FIGURING OUT FIBROMYALGIA

Current science and the most effective treatments

GINEVRA LIPTAN, M.D.

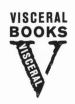

VISCERAL
BOOKS

VISCERAL
BOOKS

Figuring Out Fibromyalgia: Current Science and the Most Effective
Treatments

Published by Visceral Books, LLC
PO Box 10744
Portland, OR 97296

Visit our website: www.visceralbooks.com

First edition Jan. 2011

Book and cover design by Visible Logic, Inc. (www.visiblelogic.com)
Cover photo by Brian McDonnell
Illustrations by Bonnie Hofkin

For Dad

TABLE OF CONTENTS

INTRODUCTION:
THE F-WORD OF MEDICINE

When I developed fibromyalgia in medical school, I desperately wanted to figure out what was going on in my body. I turned to the medical experts who were my professors, and to the many medical textbooks available to me. But I was not able to find many answers—and I was horrified to learn that many doctors didn't even believe in this illness. One day during teaching rounds, as I was struggling daily with fatigue and muscle aches, one of my senior physicians authoritatively announced: "Fibromyalgia does not exist."

Although it's estimated that more than six million Americans have fibromyalgia, it remains a controversial and poorly understood diagnosis. For almost 100 years, doctors have been arguing about whether it was a "real" illness. It has gone through at least five name changes, reflecting the confusion surrounding the nature of this illness. There are still doctors that insist fibromyalgia is not real, even though there are thousands of studies documenting that it is. A recent article in *The New York Times* cast doubt on the diagnosis and quoted a leading researcher who said that fibromyalgia is not an illness; it is just "a response to stress, depression, economic, and social anxiety."[1]

The uncertainty surrounding the cause of fibromyalgia, along with a lack of effective treatments, makes this illness particularly frustrating for doctors. I have seen fibromyalgia described in medical journals as "perplexing," "mysterious," and "confusing." Informally, I have heard doctors say much worse, which is why I half-seriously refer to fibromyalgia as the F-word of medicine.

It is still regarded by some healthcare professionals as a wastebasket or catch-all diagnosis, not a specific disease. Fibromyalgia is often treated like a second-class diagnosis. No other word in medicine can evoke such a negative reaction among physicians. In a survey of doctors, fibromyalgia was rated as the least prestigious illness to treat, with heart attacks ranked as the most prestigious.[2] Some rheumatologists actually refuse to see patients for fibromyalgia. Can you imagine a doctor refusing to see someone with diabetes or high blood pressure?

Most medical providers do actually want to help, but are frustrated because they have so few tools in their toolbox. I have known this frustration as both a patient and a doctor.

I experienced first-hand how little conventional Western medicine had to offer patients with fibromyalgia. My doctor recommended exercise and anti-depressants, both of which helped me. But the exhaustion and pain continued, so I kept searching for something—anything—to feel better. Like many others with fibromyalgia, I was left to try to figure it out myself.

People with fibromyalgia tell me how tired they are of being their own doctor. One patient told me about spending $10,000 a year on alternative therapies in a wasted effort to feel better. Another described how tired she became of going to different doctors who "draw a gallon of blood, run lots of tests, and then tell me there is nothing wrong with me."

I struggled through the mass of so-called cures and supplements available on the Internet and in books. But there were so many conflicting theories being promoted, most of which seemed to be based on little if any actual scientific evidence. I saw acupuncturists, chiropractors, and naturopaths, all of whom had different ideas about the causes of fibromyalgia and how to treat it. I didn't know who to believe, and there was little scientific research to guide my decisions. So I spent years trying various alternative treatments in a very haphazard process of trial and error. This was frustrating and expensive, and I wasted huge amounts of money on ineffective treatments. The lack of guidance and answers from my doctors was frustrating.

Other people with fibromyalgia have similar feelings. A survey of almost 3,000 people with fibromyalgia found that nearly half had consulted between three and six health care providers before obtaining the diagnosis, and 25 percent had seen more than six providers prior to diagnosis. About one third of the respondents felt that their health care provider did not view fibromyalgia as a "very legitimate" disorder.[3]

Ultimately I was able to find a few alternative and experimental therapies that helped me a great deal, but only after a very expensive and agonizing process of trial and error. I was essentially studying fibromyalgia by using myself as a guinea pig. As I continued my medical training, I was able to better assess the thousands of medical studies and articles written about fibromyalgia. I began to put together why certain treatments had helped me so much, while others did nothing at all.

Over the past decade, the amount of research in fibromyalgia has increased exponentially, along with its acceptance as a legitimate medical condition. We now can document many definite, measurable abnormalities in fibromyalgia, and I review these in detail in this book. But confusion remains because many of these findings are not obvious and have to be examined in very specific ways.

Major gaps remain in our scientific understanding of this complex illness. Most importantly, we have not yet explained why it is that the muscles hurt in fibromyalgia. My personal and clinical experiences with treating this illness, along with years of studying medical research, have provided me with evidence to try to fill in this piece of the puzzle.

I am convinced that the fascia, the connective tissue surrounding each muscle, generates fibromyalgia pain. There is emerging science from many areas of research about the fascia as an important source of musculoskeletal pain, and the first scientific conference dedicated to research in this field was held at Harvard in 2007.

Part I of this book details what we currently know about fibromyalgia, along with evidence supporting the role of fascia in causing pain. The chain reaction of biological processes that leads to inflamed and painful fascia in fibromyalgia is outlined step-by-step. After reading this section you will have a better understanding of fibromyalgia than many doctors.

Part II guides you to using treatments that reduce the negative effects of each step of this chain reaction. We have not yet figured out how to stop or reverse the original trigger, but we can reduce the impact of each of the resulting problems, which can result in significant improvement in symptoms. You will also learn more about effective treatments and the science behind them.

In the third section, I review which alternative medical treatments have some evidence supporting their effectiveness and which may be a waste of money. I outline which medications can help in fibromyalgia. My involvement in medical research and treatment of fibromyalgia in a teaching hospital has enabled me to learn about new and experimental treatments.

The final chapters address some common misunderstandings and detail the rocky relationship between Western medicine and fibromyalgia.

My goal for this book is to translate complex medical information into useful guidance on effective treatments. I hope to give you a solid scientific understanding of what causes fibromyalgia so that you can use that information to help yourself feel better.

Unfortunately, because most conventional doctors have limited information and tools to use for fibromyalgia, patients often end up searching the Internet and bookstores, or blindly trying multiple alternative health therapies. Understanding more about the science of fibromyalgia will enable you to find truly effective treatments from both conventional and alternative medicine and not waste your time and money on ineffective treatments.

A decade of studying fibromyalgia and experimenting on myself has helped me to learn a lot about this mysterious illness. I don't claim to have all the answers, but I have figured out enough to experience impressive improvement in my own symptoms. While I am not "cured" of fibromyalgia, I only have about 10 percent of the pain and fatigue that I used to experience, and I have my life back.

This book is my attempt to share everything I have learned in my unique position as a physician studying fibromyalgia from the inside. It is written with the hope that my personal and professional experience with fibromyalgia can help you feel better, too.

PART I

THE CHAIN REACTION THAT CAUSES FIBROMYALGIA

1

OVERVIEW OF FIBROMYALGIA

What are the symptoms of fibromyalgia?

Frida Kahlo, an early 20th century Mexican artist, is thought to have suffered from fibromyalgia.[1] She painted a self-portrait with multiple nails piercing her entire body, which is a pretty accurate depiction of how the illness feels. People with fibromyalgia describe feeling as if they the have the flu all the time, with profound muscle pain, achiness, and fatigue. Repetitive motion tends to make the muscle pain worse. Sleep is unrefreshing, and people describe waking up in the morning feeling as if they had run a marathon overnight.

During my sickest time, I remember a deep ache all over my body. I felt so weak and tired I couldn't even lift my arms to wash my own hair. Every morning I felt exhausted and as if all my muscles had stiffened into concrete overnight.

The most common symptoms in a survey of more than 2,500 people with fibromyalgia were unrefreshing sleep, morning stiffness, fatigue, muscle pain, and problems with concentration and memory.[2] One of the most troubling symptoms is "fibrofog," a term used to describe the poor memory, reduced attention span, and difficulty multi-tasking that almost everyone with fibromyalgia experiences to some degree.

While it is usually persistent pain or fatigue that brings someone with fibromyalgia to the doctor for evaluation, there are other symptoms as well. The most common are irritable bowel and bladder symptoms, low blood pressure, dizziness on standing, and poor balance. Other symptoms can include frequent headaches, numbness or tingling in hands or feet, and sensitivity to loud noises. More information about the causes of these symptoms of fibromyalgia, and how to reduce them, are discussed further in later chapters.

About 70 percent of fibromyalgia patients have enough bowel symptoms to be diagnosed with irritable bowel syndrome, a poorly understood condition characterized by irregular bowel habits, abdominal pain, and alternating bouts of constipation and diarrhea.[3] Some fibromyalgia patients also describe symptoms of bladder discomfort as well as urgency and frequency of urination. When severe urinary symptoms are present, this condition is called interstitial cystitis, which is characterized by constant pressure and pain in the bladder along with urgency or frequency of urination. Irritable bowel and bladder symptoms also occur in people who do not have fibromyalgia, but you will learn in Chapter 8 how and why they occur with such frequency in fibromyalgia.

How is fibromyalgia diagnosed?

If you see your doctor for fatigue or muscle pain, the work-up usually starts with lab tests for thyroid function, red blood cell count, and inflammation in the blood. Muscle pain and fatigue, the main symptoms of fibromyalgia, overlap with those of many other conditions, including hypothyroidism, anemia, and some autoimmune diseases. Therefore, doctors try to rule out any other potential causes of these symptoms before making a diagnosis of fibromyalgia. All the standard laboratory tests are normal in fibromyalgia, so it often has been considered a diagnosis of exclusion, given only after no other possible cause of muscle pain and fatigue have been found.

The lack of specific lab abnormalities associated with fibromyalgia, and the fact that people don't "look sick," has contributed to the controversies surrounding this illness. Technically, fibromyalgia is not even considered a disease; it is referred to as a "syndrome." A syndrome is a collection of signs, symptoms, and medical problems that tend to occur together but are not related to a specific, identifiable cause. A "disease" is defined by having a specific cause or causes and recognizable signs and symptoms. As you will learn, I do feel that there is a specific cause for fibromyalgia, thus I do refer to it as a disease or illness throughout this book.

The lack of abnormal lab tests made diagnosing and studying this illness very difficult for many years. So in 1990, a large group of rheumatologists met and created a set of diagnostic criteria for fibromyalgia. This means that the diagnosis is based solely on symptoms and a physical exam.[4] In order to be officially diagnosed with fibromyalgia, you must have a history of diffuse musculoskeletal pain and tenderness on palpation (applied pressure) in 11 of 18 designated points.

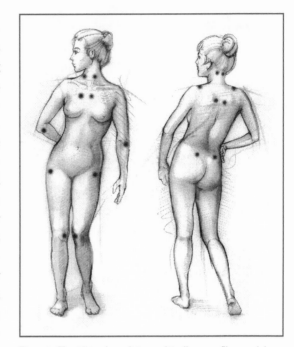

Figure 1: The 18 tender points used to diagnose fibromyalgia.

The 18 tender points used to diagnose fibromyalgia are in the muscle or tendons. The points are illustrated in Figure 1, and are on both sides of the body, just under the knees and elbows, in the low back and gluteal region, and in the neck and over the second ribs, near the breast bone.

People with fibromyalgia are usually sore in other muscles and tendons, not just the 18 designated tender points. Researchers chose those particular areas because they were found to be the most consistently tender in people with fibromyalgia, and not tender in healthy individuals. To meet the strict criteria for a fibromyalgia diagnosis, a person must have 11 or more of these tender points. This is not a perfect test, however, and some people with fibromyalgia will have fewer than 11 tender points, especially men.

Although only muscle pain and tenderness is required to make a diagnosis, fatigue and poor sleep almost always accompanies the muscle pain.

One large study found that 95 percent of fibromyalgia patients reported poor sleep quality and persistent fatigue.[5]

While most people with fibromyalgia also have unrefreshing sleep, fatigue, and memory difficulties, muscle pain is the only symptom that is currently used for diagnosis. There are researchers working on changing this and developing new diagnostic criteria that capture more of the complete picture of this illness.[6]

Who gets fibromyalgia?

Fibromyalgia affects between 2–3 percent of the U.S. population, with similar numbers worldwide. That means between six and 10 million people in the United States have fibromyalgia; more than lupus, multiple sclerosis, and Parkinson's disease combined.[7, 8] Fibromyalgia predominantly affects women; only about 10 percent of those diagnosed are men. However, in my clinical experience, it seems the proportion of men is probably a bit higher than that, making up about 15–20 percent of the fibromyalgia population.

The typical person who develops fibromyalgia is an otherwise healthy young woman in her twenties or thirties. While it usually affects people in this age range, I have diagnosed it in teenagers and in 80-year-olds. Symptoms tend to develop gradually over a few months, and often begin after a trauma such as a car accident. Nearly half of all fibromyalgia patients report that their symptoms developed within six months after a traumatic event, such as a fall, car accident, or physical assault. The association between trauma and development of fibromyalgia is discussed more in Chapter 3.

There seems to be a genetic tendency towards developing fibromyalgia. A clustering of this illness in families has been described—close relatives of people with fibromyalgia are eight times more likely to have fibromyalgia themselves.[9] Fibromyalgia is also more common in people who have system-wide inflammatory disorders such as systemic lupus erythematosus.[10]

Is it a "real" illness?

Fibromyalgia is real. Contrary to common understanding, it actually does have abnormal test findings. These are usually only seen on certain specialized tests that are primarily used for research purposes, not routine medical care. Abnormalities can be seen with specialized blood tests that look for certain markers of immune system activity. Chemicals important in transmission of pain signals are elevated in the fluid surrounding the spinal cord in fibromyalgia. Scans of blood flow in the brain reveal abnormalities in pain and stress processing areas of the brain. All of these abnormalities are subtle and complex, and are not commonly tested. This has made understanding this illness, even for medical professionals, very difficult.

In the past decade, advances in medical imaging have enabled researchers to demonstrate definite abnormalities in fibromyalgia. For the most part, this has put to rest the longstanding argument as to whether fibromyalgia actually exists. However, the cause of fibromyalgia remains a controversial and active area of research.

Part of the challenge in figuring out fibromyalgia is that it does not fit well into any one medical specialty. It was originally grouped into rheumatology, the field of medicine that treats arthritis-related disease. Arthritis refers to inflammation of the joints, which is not actually seen in fibromyalgia. "Fibromyalgia is very different from other rheumatological diseases, probably because it isn't a rheumatologic disease," says Dr. M. Catherine Bushnell.[11] Fibromyalgia actually straddles the specialties of sleep medicine, neurology (brain and nerves), and endocrinology (hormones). It is a bit of an orphan illness, without a specific specialty to call home.

History of fibromyalgia

The confusion surrounding fibromyalgia is illustrated by the multiple names given to this condition over the past 200 years. A syndrome of widespread muscle pain and fatigue was first described in the early 19th century, and called either "chronic rheumatism" or "muscular rheumatism," but was incorrectly attributed to a bacterial infection. Dr. Ralph Stockman described the symptoms of chronic rheumatism as "pain, aching, stiffness, a readiness to feel muscular fatigue, interference with free muscular movement, and very often a want of energy and vigour."[12]

In 1904, during a now famous lecture at a London hospital, Sir William Gowers proposed that chronic rheumatism was caused by inflammation of the fibrous tissue surrounding muscles. He suggested that the condition be called "fibrositis," and that term was used until the 1970s.[13] The use of this term reflected the belief that the immune system was attacking the muscles and causing inflammation. But after years of research, no scientific evidence of muscle inflammation was found, so the term was replaced by "fibromyalgia." The current name contains the Latin words for fiber, muscle, and pain.

What medical science knows about fibromyalgia—a brief overview

Over the past decade researchers have established dysfunction in sleep, pain, and the stress response in fibromyalgia. Of course, even with all the current objective evidence of abnormalities in fibromyalgia, there are still doctors who don't believe it's real. A Harvard-trained neurologist recently told me he thought it was "just a behavioral disorder."

However, if your doctor were to read an article in a major medical journal about fibromyalgia, the following points might be discussed:

- **Abnormalities of the stress response**
  The nervous system has two ways to respond to stress, and dysfunction in both those systems have been described in fibromyalgia. One simple way to think of this is that the stress response gets stuck in the "fight-or-flight" mode in fibromyalgia.

- **Disrupted sleep**
  Many studies have noted abnormalities in sleep in fibromyalgia. The major abnormality observed is a reduction in the amount and quality of deep sleep. Abnormal brain waves frequently interrupt deep sleep in fibromyalgia patients, resulting in poor sleep that is non-restorative.

- **Low growth hormone levels**
  In adulthood, growth hormone is responsible for regulating the repair and maintenance of muscle and is primarily secreted dur-

ing deep sleep and after exercise. Multiple studies have shown that patients with fibromyalgia have inadequate growth hormone release.

- **Pain processing**

  There is dysfunction of the pain-processing systems in fibromyalgia. Studies show that the nervous system is hyper-reactive to stimuli. So pain hurts more, hot is hotter, loud is louder, etc. This process is called central sensitization. You can think of it as a nervous system that is turning up the volume on any input it receives.

This is just a very brief overview of our scientific understanding of these problems. In the following chapters you will learn much more about the stress response, sleep, and pain processing in fibromyalgia. You will also learn how these problems interact in a chain reaction that ultimately results in muscle pain and fatigue. There are some very large gaps in current medical understanding of fibromyalgia, and you will learn about cutting-edge research that is filling in these gaps.

And most importantly, you will learn how to lessen the impact of each step in this chain reaction to reduce your own symptoms.

2

MY STORY

At the end of my first year of medical school, I was doing crunches at the gym when I felt a muscle in the front of my neck rip. I had never heard of anyone pulling a muscle in the *front* of the neck. But I had pulled other muscles before, and I figured this would heal right up. But as days turned to weeks, it didn't get better. It felt like my neck was tired of holding the weight of my head. The only relief I got was when I wrapped a heating pad around my neck.

I saw a chiropractor who found some mild abnormalities in my cervical spine and did some adjustments to my neck. I started getting regular chiropractic adjustments, because they were all I could think to do, and they did help reduce my neck pain a little.

Over the summer, I started to feel achy and tired all the time. I took a part-time baby-sitting job, and after working for just a few hours I was exhausted for days. I woke up in the morning with a sore neck and back, which hurt all day. I frequently felt stiff, weak, and lightheaded, as though I was 100 years old. It felt like all the energy of my body and mind had been sucked out. A constant, dull ache developed near my ear that got worse when I chewed or yawned. I did some research on my own and realized I had developed the symptoms of temporomandibular joint dysfunction (TMD).

I went to see my doctor, who prescribed a muscle relaxant and suggested I might be grinding my teeth at night, a common cause of TMD pain. I saw a dentist, who said my teeth showed no evidence of grinding. He couldn't find any dental causes for my jaw pain. The muscle relaxant did not help at all.

As the summer wore on the pain progressed to my upper back; an ache between my shoulder blades that would not go away. I woke every morning as one big ache. It felt like my spine hurt, my skin hurt, everything hurt. I was sleeping poorly, tossing and turning, and I awoke every morning feeling more tired than before I went to bed. I felt too weak to even lift my arms up to wash my hair in the shower.

One day my hips started aching, so much that I couldn't do anything but lie in bed and cry. I was sure there was something really wrong with me, so I went to see my primary care doctor. She drew blood tests and sent me to a rheumatologist. The rheumatologist ordered x-rays of my neck and hips and assured me they were completely normal. "So why do I hurt all the time?" I asked. His response was, "I don't know, but you don't have arthritis."

I returned to my primary doctor to find that my labs were all normal. My doctors had no answers for me and nothing to offer.

A diagnosis

I started my second year of medical school as a total wreck. And then a bit of grace fell my way. My chiropractor sold her practice. After telling my entire story to the new chiropractor, he suggested for the first time that I might have fibromyalgia. He checked my tender points, and I had exquisite tenderness in at least 10 of the points. He recommended that I read what he called "the bible of fibromyalgia," *Fibromyalgia and Chronic Myofascial Pain Syndrome: A Survival Manual*.

I spent weeks reading and rereading this book, trying to convince myself that I did not have fibromyalgia. I fluctuated between being relieved that what I was experiencing had a name, and denial that it was indeed my illness. The description of symptoms did sound like me, but denial is a powerful force. My mind jumped on every symptom mentioned in the book that I was not experiencing: *Aha! See I don't have fibromyalgia*. It felt like a death sentence to me. "Chronic" was such an awful word. And fibromyalgia had such a stigma among doctors—even among my fellow medical students—that I really didn't want to believe I had it. My intellectual battle continued.

Endless Research

I began intensely researching fibromyalgia in my medical textbooks, on the Internet, and in bookstores. The search was completely overwhelming. It seemed Western medicine had little to offer as far as understanding this mysterious illness, and the only treatments available were antidepressants and regular exercise. I was already on antidepressants and was exercising as much as I could, but still felt awful.

So I ventured into the confusing world of alternative medicine. On the Internet I read countless theories and suggested treatments for fibromyalgia, many of which conflicted directly with what I was learning in medical school. Since Western medicine didn't seem to have any solutions, though, I felt compelled to try alternative treatments. But what should I do? I was overwhelmed by the different theories I encountered about the cause of fibromyalgia and how to treat it:

- Is it yeast overgrowth causing symptoms? Should I try prescription anti-fungals and a strict low sugar diet?

- Do I need to cleanse my body of toxins? Should I do a raw juice fast?

- Is it low thyroid? Do I need to get my thyroid checked with a special test, not the standard one doctors use? And if so, how am I going to pay for it since I'm not working and my insurance won't cover it?

- Should I use guaifenesin to reduce calcium phosphate deposits in the muscles?

- Am I deficient is some vitamin that I need to take mega-doses of?

- Is it all just caused by stress and is daily meditation the answer?

- Do I need to eat macrobiotically? Only raw foods? Only alkaline foods?

Compounding my confusion and frustration was the fact that I was so fatigued. I didn't have the resources or the energy to get expensive tests done or begin a special diet. I tried acupuncture for a few months—no help—and massage, which seemed to make me feel more achy and tired.

In the midst of all this confusion, I met another medical student dealing with similar health problems. She had experienced improvement after getting alternative treatments for yeast overgrowth and toxicity, so she recommended I try colonics and fasting to rid my body of toxins. Having never heard of colonics, she described them to me in great, gory detail: The procedure involves having a tube inserted into your rectum, and gently flushing the colon with warm water, and then allowing the flushed material to flow out the tube.

I was disgusted and a bit freaked out, but she swore by them and said they had helped her, and that they were a great way to decrease toxins in the body. I spent the rest of that fall cleansing and fasting and getting colonics. I read books that proclaimed toxicity as the cause of all illness. I followed the body ecology diet, which advocated a low-sugar vegetarian diet and eating only certain types of foods that were not acidic.

The frequent deprivation made me feel sorry for myself, and with the stress of that fall I fell right back into binging on the forbidden sugar. After a massive sugar binge, I would come back with more resolve to eat no sugar, drink my algae shakes three times a day, and get colonics more often. I would then fast for days, eating nothing but raw vegetable juice.

I bounced around like that all fall, but I wasn't feeling any better. In fact I was feeling worse, weaker, and definitely poorer. At $60 per session, colonics were not cheap. I was depressed, stressed, and still felt terrible.

Not convinced of my own toxicity

I spent much of my second year of medical school trying to detoxify myself. My heart was never really in it, but it had helped my friend. I estimate that I spent at least $8,000 on unsuccessful detoxification treatments, and I actually felt worse.

I was beating my head against the wall, trying to cleanse my body of its toxicity, its badness, its dirtiness. *Purify! Fast! Colonics! Not feeling better yet? It is because you are still toxic and need to do more fasting with even harsher restrictions.*

I finally gave up on the idea that toxicity in my body was causing my symptoms. It didn't really make sense to me. Everyone's living on this same toxic planet, but not everyone is sick. My husband eats, drinks, and breathes what I do, but he is not sick. I never felt a good explanation for *why* being toxic would cause my neck to ache.

The latter half of my second year of medical school was basically a very expensive correspondence course. I rarely felt well enough to make it to class, and survived by getting lecture notes from friends, studying at home, and showing up only for the occasional required seminar and for exams. I began to realize that there was no way I could make it through the rigors of third year medical school, with 80-hour work weeks and high levels of physical and emotional stress.

So I made plans to take leave of absence. My hope was to devote this time to working on my health. Financially though, I still had to work. The woman who ran the colonics clinic offered to train and hire me to do colonics at the clinic. I accepted, against my better judgment. Colonics hadn't really helped my health at all, but it excited me to be working in a holistic health environment and I thought I might learn something from being there. Plus it was a paying job!

I crawled across the finish line of my second year, and starting training on administering colonics. I had not realized that colonics are actually fairly physically demanding to administer. While one hand holds the tubing in place so does not slide out of the rectum, the other hand massages the abdomen and holds pressure on various points.

After only a few weeks on the job, I started to notice my forearms ached when I came home from work. The ache progressed to a burning numbness in my forearms and fingers. My thumb joint began throbbing. I tried changing my position frequently at work, I tried stretching before work, but the pain in my arms and hands persisted. My arms felt so weak I couldn't lift a dish to wash it without excruciating pain. I realized that I had to quit this job. I gave my notice after working there for only a few months.

I was now jobless, and in such constant arm pain that any movement was difficult. How was I supposed to work at *any* job, let alone finish medical school? How would I ever be able to pay back my already substantial student loan debt? My health was worse now then at the beginning of the year, and I didn't see how I could possibly return to school in a few months.

Looking for Hope

I finally accepted that I had fibromyalgia. I felt hopeless and helpless. I kept telling myself that this was not fatal and it was not cancer, but it felt like a death sentence to be 26 years old and feel like you were 100.

But I had a really hard time accepting that it was chronic and incurable. Even in my darkest times, I thought there had to be a way that I could feel better. I just needed to find it. What gave me hope was hearing that others had gotten better.

I remember one particularly low moment, desperately searching the Internet with my husband. In tears I told him, "I just need to know that one person got better, that it's *possible*." And at that exact moment he clicked on a website selling a book entitled *Fibromyalgia: How I Recovered Completely*. We both burst out laughing. I ordered the book and felt my hope returning.

But the book that really helped me was Claire Musickant's *Fibromyalgia: My Journey to Wellness*. In it she describes her great success with using blood allergy testing. I knew it was something I needed to do; it felt right. I felt a rush of excitement as I called the lab that administered the test to find a practitioner in my area. I was given the name of a naturopath. I called her and found out the test would cost more than $300. I hesitated and asked her if it had helped people with fibromyalgia in her experience. "Oh yes," she said, "and it helped me. I had fibromyalgia and am now 90 percent better."

She *had* fibromyalgia—*past tense*. These were possibly the most beautiful words I had ever heard. She was the first person I had talked to that had even suggested that fibromyalgia was something one could get better from. Now I had not only read the stories of two people recovering, but I had also actually talked to a real live person who had gotten better!

Results

After the results of my blood testing came back, I still was not convinced this could help me, but I was desperate enough to try anything. I started to avoid the foods and chemicals in my diet according to the test results. After about two weeks, I realized that the all-over body ache I had grown so accustomed to was gone. It didn't feel as if I constantly had the flu. I had the energy to grocery shop, to cook, to exercise.

I was very encouraged and kept up the routine for the next year and a half. I went from actively aching all the time to only hurting when someone pressed on my muscles, and feeling less exhausted. But I still struggled with neck and arm pain, and it seemed any exertion or repeated motion really made me hurt.

Later that year I stumble across a manual therapy called myofascial release (MFR) that really helped my arm and neck pain. It was recommended to me by a massage therapist as a treatment "that helps with fibromyalgia."

MFR is a therapy involving slow, prolonged stretching of the muscles. These stretches release restrictions in the fascia, the connective tissue around the muscle (see Chapter 11 for further details). I found this therapy to be incredibly helpful for my muscle pain.

I was well enough to return to medical school, and I began studying fibromyalgia, trying to figure out how and why the blood allergy testing and myofascial release helped me. I finished medical school and a rigorous residency in internal medicine, regularly working 80-hour weeks.

Today I still have fibromyalgia, but feel about 90 percent better than I did at first. I describe more about my experiences with various treatments—and the science behind them—in the following chapters.

3

FIBROMYALGIA
AS A CHAIN REACTION

Research indicates that fibromyalgia involves a malfunction in the stress and pain response systems of the body. After reading this chapter, you will be an expert on both of these subjects. This information is available in the medical literature, but not in a way that is easily accessible or understandable to the layperson trying to learn about fibromyalgia.

Chronic over-activation of the stress response in the brain starts a chain reaction leading to poor deep sleep, muscle pain, and fatigue. Ultimately, all the symptoms of fibromyalgia stem from abnormal activation of the fight-or-flight nervous system. In the next few chapters, I will walk you through the biological processes that result from a nervous system stuck in the fight-or-flight response.

Deep sleep is inhibited because the brain is trying to stay alert to fend off danger. A lack of deep sleep causes fatigue and prevents adequate growth hormone release. A lack of growth hormone interferes with the normal muscle tissue repair process and leads to muscle pain. Muscles and their surrounding connective tissue are chronically tightened to respond to danger and become painful.

The pain signals streaming up to the brain from muscles overwhelm the nervous system and cause it to become hyper-reactive to pain. The nervous system starts interpreting pain signals incorrectly, and even just a light touch of the skin may be experienced as pain.

The Chain Reaction Of Fibromyalgia

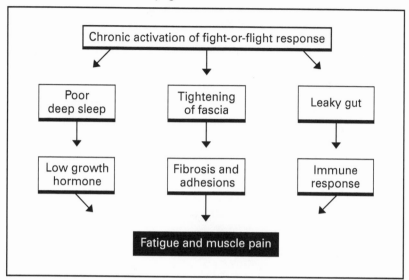

Fight or Flight

The chain reaction of fibromyalgia starts deep in the brain, in the area that controls the body's emergency response system to stress. This does not mean "stress" as we commonly use it in conversation, as in, "I'm so stressed out." The stress response in the scientific sense is the body's automatic response to any real or perceived danger.

The stress response is the body's alarm reaction. It is not under conscious control; it is controlled deep in the primal parts of the brain. You don't have to think about responding to stress. It is a reflex, the same type of automatic response as pulling your hand away from a hot stove. The response to stress is so automatic that it even happens when people are in a coma or under sedation for surgery. According to Dr. Hans Selye, a pioneer in the field, "Stress can be produced under deep anesthesia in patients who are unconscious, and even in cell cultures grown outside the body."[1]

The hypothalamus, a gland deep in the brain, directs the stress response. When danger is sensed it signals the adrenal glands to produce adrenaline, which acts to prepare the body for emergency action. If you have ever been startled by a loud noise, causing your heart to pound, you have experienced the effects of a massive adrenaline release.

Along with regulating the release of adrenaline, the hypothalamus controls the autonomic nervous system. This is the main system of the body in charge of regulating essential functions such as blood pressure, heart rate, breathing, digestion, and urination. One way to think about the autonomic nervous system is as the autopilot that controls the housekeeping operations of the body. It is not under conscious control—you don't have to think about digesting your food, your body does it automatically. The autopilot nervous system has two simple modes, one designed for times of safety and one designed for times of danger or stress.

These two modes have opposing functions, like the accelerator and brake in your car. When a threat is perceived, the hypothalamus pushes the accelerator and activates the adrenal glands and the sympathetic nervous system. When no danger is sensed, the hypothalamus puts on the brake and activates the parasympathetic nervous system.

Actions of the Autonomic Nervous System

Sympathetic activation (the accelerator)	Parasympathetic activation (the brake)
Pupil dilation	Pupil constriction
Heart rate and force increased	Heart rate and force decreased
Blood flow diverted away from GI system	Blood flow increases to GI system
Reduced gastric secretions and digestion	Increased gastric secretion and digestions
Slower gastric motility	Faster gastric motility
Blood vessels constricted	Blood vessels relaxed
Muscles tensed	Muscles relaxed

To remember the difference, every medical student memorizes that the sympathetic nervous system readies the body for "fight-or-flight" action and the parasympathetic promotes a "rest-and-digest" mode. Imagine a cave-woman curled up around a fire in her cave. Her muscles are relaxed and at rest. Her digestive system is busy processing dinner, her heart rate is slow, and she feels warm and sleepy. Her autopilot nervous system is in the rest-and-digest mode.

Now imagine the same cavewoman suddenly spots a saber-toothed tiger at the entrance to her cave. The fight-or-flight mode of the autopilot nervous system kicks in, and instantly her heart pounds, her muscles tense, and she is ready to fight for her life or run away. Blood flow is diverted away from non-critical functions like the digestive system, and adrenaline is pumping through her blood. Her awareness and vigilance about her surroundings increase.

In fibromyalgia, the stress response system is stuck in the fight-or flight mode because the hypothalamus is continually sending signals of imminent danger to the body. It's like a malfunctioning smoke alarm that beeps even though there is no smoke.

The stress response nervous system is complex and dynamic, but recent methods looking at variation in the heart rate can assess the level of activation of the fight-or-flight nervous system. One study monitored fibromyalgia subjects' heartbeats while they followed their routine daily activities for 24 hours and found a "relentless hyperactivity of the sympathetic nervous system" that continued even while sleeping.[2] Another study found excessive firing of sympathetic nerves to muscles in fibromyalgia.[3] Much higher blood levels of the main stress hormone of the sympathetic nervous system were observed in one study, leading the authors to conclude that "fibromyalgia may represent a primary disorder of the stress system."[4]

The fight-or-flight response is so over-activated in fibromyalgia that it becomes less able to respond to actual stressors.[5] This phenomenon is sometimes labeled "adrenal fatigue" by alternative health care practitioners, but it's better described as "adrenal inflexibility." When the accelerator pedal is pressed all the way to the floor, you can't push it down any further to get more speed. In fact, this leads to some of the other common symptoms seen in fibromyalgia, such as low blood pressure and dizziness upon standing.

Normally, going from a seated to standing position triggers the sympathetic nervous system to constrict the blood vessels in the legs to prevent a drop in blood pressure. In fibromyalgia, the sympathetic blood vessel constriction is already at maximum so cannot constrict any further. This results in the very common occurrence of low blood pressure, dizziness, or even fainting upon standing seen in fibromyalgia.[6]

Trauma and the brain

We don't know for certain exactly how or why the stress response gets stuck in the danger mode in fibromyalgia. There seems to be a genetic component; fibromyalgia tends to run in families just like diabetes and many other chronic illnesses. The most widely accepted current theory is that in genetically predisposed people, a trauma may trigger a prolonged activation of the stress response system.[7]

A fascinating brain imaging study recently found changes in the size and make up of the stress processing structures in fibromyalgia subjects.[8] While we do recognize that there may be a genetic component to developing fibromyalgia, we have not yet identified any specific gene that is to blame.

A strong association has been shown between childhood trauma or abuse and the later development of fibromyalgia. Studies estimate that more than half of women with fibromyalgia have experienced childhood sexual abuse. One study found that among a population of women diagnosed with fibromyalgia, more than 90 percent had experienced a sexual or physical assault in their lifetime.[9] There is also some overlap between fibromyalgia and another disease closely linked to trauma, post-traumatic stress disorder (PTSD). In one study, almost half of the male patients with combat-related PTSD met the diagnostic criteria for fibromyalgia.[10]

Although both PTSD and fibromyalgia are considered to be trauma-related illnesses, they are not identical. PTSD is characterized by recurrent, emotionally intense traumatic memories, nightmares, and avoidance behaviors. Brain imaging reveals dysfunction in the amygdala and hippocampus, areas of the brain that are important in the emotional memory and fear systems of the brain.[11]

Either PTSD or fibromyalgia might develop after a trauma, depending on which areas of the brain are affected. In fibromyalgia, the dysfunction is in the fight-or-flight response, whereas in PTSD the fear-response areas of the brain are affected. Certainly, all of these areas can be affected in one individual, and many people with fibromyalgia also have PTSD.

A trauma to the developing brain may set the stage for development of fibromyalgia in adulthood. Traumas in childhood or adolescence can be potent triggers of an abnormal and prolonged stress response. The growing and developing brain is more strongly affected by trauma. The brains of rats exposed to stress during puberty show more changes in the stress-response areas compared to rats exposed to the exact same stress as adults.[12]

Even for those who have experienced childhood trauma, sometimes the symptoms of fibromyalgia do not develop until after a second trauma in adulthood. Some people do not identify any childhood trauma, but experience a car accident, attack, or major illness or surgery as an adult that seems to trigger fibromyalgia. One study reported that "physical trauma in the preceding six months is significantly associated with the onset of fibromyalgia."[13] It is estimated that between 25–50 percent of patients report a physical trauma in the six months preceding the onset of their fibromyalgia.[14, 15]

While most people with fibromyalgia can identify a trauma in childhood or adulthood—or both—not everyone does. So there are some alternate theories about how the stress response system can be triggered. In some people with fibromyalgia, intermittent or constant spinal cord compression in the neck may be causing or promoting sympathetic nervous system over-activity. Spinal cord impingement may activate or irritate the sympathetic nervous system. Anything that irritates the spinal cord in the neck could potentially trigger a prolonged activation of the fight-or-flight response.

The Chiari malformation, a rare congenital abnormality where the base of the brain protrudes into the spinal canal, has been suggested as a potential irritant to the spinal cord in fibromyalgia. Another theory is that spinal cord compression from herniated disks or a narrow spinal column in the neck could provoke fibromyalgia symptoms. Two interesting studies found a high rate of cervical cord compression in fibromyalgia patients, but only when the neck was in certain positions.[16, 17] However, other studies have found that Chiari malformations and cervical cord compressions occur at the same rates in both healthy people as in people with fibromyalgia.[18]

A very experienced nurse practitioner that I work with who studies this topic feels that for a small group of people with fibromyalgia, spinal cord compression in the neck may be a significant contributing factor. She has had a few patients whose fibromyalgia symptoms dramatically improved after pressure on their spinal cord was relieved with specialized physical therapy or surgery.

While this remains an active area of research, it is not clear if there is a connection between cervical cord compression and activation of the fight-or-flight system in fibromyalgia. Any thorough fibromyalgia evaluation should include a physical examination looking for signs of spinal cord compression of the neck, which can include abnormal reflexes or weakness of the arms.

Sleep pattern abnormalities

When the nervous system gets stuck in the fight-or-flight mode, it has negative affects on the body, especially in regards to sleep. Imagine if the saber-toothed tiger stayed at our cave woman's cave entrance 24 hours a day. If she were able to sleep with a tiger at her door, would she get restful sleep? No, she would be sleeping very lightly, be hyper-vigilant with all her body's alarm systems still on, ready to run away or fight for her life at any moment.

The hypothalamus in fibromyalgia is stuck in the fight-or-flight mode even while sleeping. As you can imagine, if the brain and nervous system are always in emergency, survival mode, this would be a potent inhibitor of deep sleep. It would be like trying to park your car while pressing the accelerator.

One patient told me she felt like she "sleeps with one eye open." So someone with fibromyalgia awakens feeling exhausted, as if they got no sleep because even in their sleep their brain is awake and watching out for saber-toothed tigers. In surveys, nearly all of fibromyalgia patients describe their sleep as poor and not restful.[19]

Sleep studies have consistently demonstrated that fibromyalgia patients experience abnormal sleep cycles with reduced and interrupted deep sleep. Deep sleep in fibromyalgia is frequently interrupted by brain waves normally seen only while awake.[20] Studies also show that activation of the fight-or-flight nervous system at night causes excessive arousal and awakening episodes and the inability to get prolonged deep sleep seen in fibromyalgia.[21]

The symptoms of fibromyalgia can be induced in healthy people by simply depriving them of deep sleep. A pioneering 1975 study was able to induce widespread muscle pain in healthy college students after a few nights of interrupting their deep sleep with loud sounds. These symptoms went away after a few nights of normal sleep.

In fibromyalgia, the brain itself is sending an arousal signal—an alpha brain wave—each time deep sleep is reached and jolting the brain back to a lighter stage of sleep. But the end result is the same: interrupted and inadequate deep sleep, fatigue, and achiness.[22]

Normal human sleep consists of different cycles of brain and body activity throughout the night, and each phase of sleep has unique functions. The most important phase of sleep for the body is called deep sleep. This is when the body is motionless and brain waves are very slow. This stage is what makes you fell rested the next day, and is the time when your body does very important housekeeping and repair processes, like janitors coming in each night to empty the wastebaskets and vacuum to get ready for the next day.

Many people confuse deep sleep with rapid eye movement sleep (REM), but they are very different. During REM sleep, your brain is actively processing information into dreams and is not communicating much with the body. During deep sleep, the brain is not processing information, but is quietly sending signals throughout the body to direct housekeeping and repair operations. One of the most important repair signals sent out by the brain during deep sleep is growth hormone. If deprived of deep sleep, not enough growth hormone is released, and this can lead to poor tissue repair and muscle pain.

Low growth hormone levels

Lack of deep sleep not only leads to fatigue, it also affects the body's ability to heal. The key element here is the production of growth hormone, most of which occurs during deep sleep.[23] Some other triggers of growth hormone release include exercise and high-protein meals.

Multiple studies have found low growth hormone levels in fibromyalgia. One study measured lower levels of growth hormone release over a 24-hour period, with the decrease most noticeable during the night.[24-27] People with fibromyalgia also have lower than normal growth hormone response to exercise.[28]

Growth hormone is the main regulator of growth in tissues, and low levels are problematic because this hormone is essential for muscle health.[29] As we grow taller and bigger throughout childhood, this hormone orchestrates the remodeling and recycling of tissue that allows bones and muscles to become longer. Once we have reached our full adult height, growth hormone continues to regulate the recycling and repair of tissue.

In particular, it is very important for the repair of tiny traumas to the muscles induced by daily activity and exercise. This is why many athletes and bodybuilders use artificial growth hormone supplementation to try to increase muscle growth and speed up recovery between training sessions. Growth hormone supplementation also speeds up post-operative wound healing and healing from burns.[30, 31]

Several studies support a connection between low growth hormone levels and increased muscle pain. When given growth hormone replacement, some fibromyalgia patients had significant reduction in symptoms and muscle tenderness.[32, 33]

Abnormal pain processing

How do chronic fight-or-flight activation, interrupted deep sleep, and low growth hormone levels in fibromyalgia lead to muscle pain? This is perhaps the most complex and difficult-to-understand aspect of fibromyalgia, even for doctors. Although the muscles hurt in fibromyalgia, no one has been able to find an explanation for the muscle pain. The muscles look and act normally in fibromyalgia. This lead to doubt and skepticism as to whether fibromyalgia was real for many years.

We still have not found a widely accepted explanation as to why the muscles hurt (see Chapter 4), but we have finally been able to demonstrate with brain-imaging studies that people fibromyalgia are experiencing significant pain. These high-tech studies also showed that the brain and spinal cord in fibromyalgia are hyper-reactive to pain.

A groundbreaking study in 2002 showed that fibromyalgia subjects experienced more pain in response to thumb pressure.[34] In this study, the subject's thumb was placed in a compression device and was squeezed until the subjects said, "Ouch." During this process, researchers watched the real-time activity of blood flow in the brain. Compared to healthy individuals, people with fibromyalgia said "ouch" at much less thumb pressure. And at that point of saying "ouch," all pain-processing areas of the brain were lit up in fibromyalgia patients. The pain in fibromyalgia was finally able to be objectively measured.

The other very important finding in this study was that people with fibromyalgia experienced pain with much lighter amounts of thumb pressure. Pressures that that did not activate any pain in healthy people caused fibromyalgia subjects to experience high amounts of pain and activated pain-processing areas in the brain.

This phenomenon is called central sensitization, and is due to amplification of pain signals in the spinal cord and abnormal processing of pain signals in the brain. Essentially the spinal cord starts turning up the volume on *all* the signals it gets, including pain signals. Even light pressure is translated into a very loud pain signal in the brain. This phenomenon is not exclusive to fibromyalgia, and occurs in other chronic pain conditions. But finding central sensitization in fibromyalgia did direct research interest in how the central nervous system (brain and spinal cord) processes pain in fibromyalgia.

The technical term for this abnormal processing and amplification of pain signals is "central sensitization" or "spinal cord hyper-reactivity." It primarily occurs due to alterations of chemicals and receptors in the cells of the spinal cord, especially a chemical called Substance P that is important in the transmission of pain signals. Studies of the spinal cord fluid show three times higher Substance P levels in the spinal fluid in fibromyalgia compared to healthy controls.[35]

Imagine you touch a hot stove and burn your finger. The nerves in your skin send a pain signal to the spinal cord, which then transmits the signal to the brain, and once the signal hits your brain you feel the pain in your finger. There are pain-sensing nerves in almost every part of the body. These nerves are called peripheral nerves (because they are outside the spinal cord) and they send pain signals from the skin, muscles, bones, and organs. Information is transmitted from the nerve to the spinal cord and then to the brain. This may seem straightforward, but both the spinal cord and brain perform complex processing of that signal as it gets transmitted.

Sometimes when nerves send continual pain signals it overwhelms the processing ability of the spinal cord. Think of it as a telephone operator becoming overwhelmed by a high volume of calls, who starts transferring calls to the wrong places. The brain is not able to adequately filter this mess of pain signals, and is trying to listen to all of them. So the brain is also turning up the volume, trying to interpret the pain.

Now, at each step of the pain signal as it travels through the spinal cord into the brain, it gets a little louder. Imagine children playing the game of telephone by whispering the same word to their neighbor down the line, but each saying the word slightly louder than they heard it. What started as a whispered "*waffles*" might have transformed into "*MOTHBALLS!*" screamed into the ear of the last child.

That is in essence what the spinal cord is doing when it is hypersensitive to pain. It is taking a signal it gets from the nerves and turning up the volume on it so that by the time it gets to the brain, it is extremely loud and sounds different from the original signal. It's not just pain signals that are interpreted incorrectly by a hyper-reactive spinal cord. Messages sent up the spinal cord from the nerves that sense temperature and pressure can also be misinterpreted. This may explain the intolerance to temperature extremes or weather-related pressure changes experienced by many people with fibromyalgia.

What leads to the last step in the chain reaction?

The findings of increased pain sensitivity seen in the original 2002 study have since been confirmed in many other studies.[36] There is strong evidence that in fibromyalgia the spinal cord is amplifying and misinterpreting pain signals. This has provided validation of the diagnosis for many doctors and researchers, and directed research for medications targeting the spinal cord processing of pain. It helps explain why even just a touch of the skin can hurt and why the pain of fibromyalgia can be so debilitating and severe.

The chain reaction of fibromyalgia begins with activation of the fight-or-flight response and ends with abnormal pain processing in the spinal cord. But we are still missing a key piece of the puzzle: How do we connect chronic stress response activation, inadequate deep sleep, and low growth hormone levels to abnormal pain processing?

As you will see in the next few chapters, the fascia, or connective tissue around the muscle, may be the missing link.

4

IS FIBROMYALGIA PAIN ALL IN YOUR SPINAL CORD?

Since patients with fibromyalgia complain of sore and painful muscles, researchers have been searching for evidence of muscle disease or dysfunction for more than 100 years. However, study after study analyzing fibromyalgia muscle cells under the microscope have not revealed any abnormalities that could explain the muscle pain.[1] Muscles also function normally in fibromyalgia, which initially lead many doctors to conclude that the condition is not real, and must be due to psychological issues.

More recently, imaging studies of the brain have highlighted the amplification of pain signals seen in fibromyalgia, and has lead to acceptance that fibromyalgia pain is real. The current medical theory is that all of fibromyalgia pain can be explained by pain amplification in the spinal cord and brain, also called "central sensitization" or "spinal cord hyper-reactivity." The idea is that since the muscles appear normal in fibromyalgia, something must go haywire in the nerves and spinal cord, causing them to constantly send "false" pain signals that the muscles hurt.

But blaming all the pain on central sensitization is incomplete and does not answer two key questions:

1. Why do people with fibromyalgia hurt more in specific areas of their muscles?
2. What triggers the spinal cord amplification of pain?

It is important to understand that central sensitization is not exclusive to fibromyalgia. It is seen in many different chronic pain conditions including endometriosis, low back pain, and arthritis.[2, 3] It is actually a well-known response to chronic pain signals from any source—muscles, bone, or skin. In other chronic pain conditions, we can identify a trigger. For example, we know that irritated nerves in a joint inflamed by arthritis send out the pain signals that induce spinal cord hyper-reactivity. What we don't know is exactly where the pain signals in fibromyalgia are coming from.

A fire that starts without a spark?

To understand this process better, imagine some noisy neighbors move into the apartment below you. At first the noise doesn't bother you much, because you figure it's only going to be temporary. But it continues, day in and day out. All night long they're making a horrible racket. You start to become extremely sensitive to any noise from downstairs, listening intently to try and figure out what on earth they are doing down there.

This is what the spinal cord is doing in response to its own noisy neighbors, the peripheral nerves that are constantly sending up pain signals. So the spinal cord becomes more sensitive to pain signals it receives on a frequent basis, just as the noisy neighbor triggered you to become more sensitive to any sounds they make.

The lack of any muscle problems in fibromyalgia has lead to the conclusion that the spinal cord hyper-reactivity must just happen spontaneously—with no trigger. The research community is essentially divided into two opposing camps of thought on this topic. One groups claims that there is nothing abnormal in the muscle in fibromyalgia. The other group argues that there must be something wrong in the muscles; we just don't know what it is yet. As you can probably gather, I fall into the latter group.

I simply find it hard to believe that the well-described process of spinal cord hyper-reactivity is somehow completely different in fibromyalgia. That's a bit like looking at a fire and concluding that because you cannot find the spark that ignited it, this must be an entirely new kind of fire that starts without a spark. It seems more reasonable to assume that we simply have not yet identified the painful trigger, rather than assuming a trigger does not exist.

However, the opposing camp has a good point. We have not been able to find anything in the muscles that could be sending out pain signals. This is the huge hole in our current understanding of fibromyalgia. What is the painful input—the noisy downstairs neighbor—that triggers the spinal cord to become hyper-reactive?

Identifying the trigger

It is essential to identify what causes the central sensitization in fibromyalgia so that we can find treatments that actually address the root of the pain, not just the end effect of the pain on the spinal cord. In fact, if the constant pain signaling to the spinal cord is reduced or eliminated, the hyper-reactivity in the spinal cord calms down.

Imagine if your downstairs neighbors from hell move away. You would gradually stop listening for their noise, and would settle back into normalcy. This also happens with the spinal cord hyper-reactivity to pain. One study found that people with chronic hip pain from arthritis had developed spinal cord hyper-reactivity to pain, but this returned to normal a few months after successful joint replacement surgery.[4]

This is why it is vital to identify the painful trigger in fibromyalgia. And there are some powerful arguments that support the idea that pain signals coming from the muscles trigger the spinal cord hyper-reactivity in fibromyalgia.[5]

Most obviously, people with fibromyalgia describe pain in their muscles that is worsened after muscle exertion or overuse. This suggests a local source of pain in the muscles themselves, and is not what would be expected if the pain were coming entirely from the spinal cord.

The painful tender points used to diagnose fibromyalgia are located in the muscles and tendons at areas that suffer from the most mechanical use and tissue damage with activity. If pain was coming primarily from the spinal cord, you would expect it to be fairly evenly distributed throughout the body, not worsened in certain areas of the muscles that experience greater strain and tissue damage. Fibromyalgia pain is not evenly distributed, but is most prevalent in certain areas of the muscles, especially the shoulders, chest, and lower back.[6] Finally, the reduction in pain experienced after muscle trigger point injections supports the idea of a generator of pain located in the muscle tissue itself.

A few recent nerve studies provide even more support for the role of painful input from the muscles leading to the spinal cord hyper-reactivity in fibromyalgia.[7, 8] Injection of numbing medicine into the trapezius muscle in fibromyalgia patients actually reduced the heightened sensitivity to heat in the skin of the forearm, completely away from the site of the numbing injection. This indicates that when the painful muscle stimulus to the spinal cord was removed for even a brief time, the spinal cord was able to calm down a bit and process signals like temperature more correctly.

Studies have shown that the muscle cells look and act normally in fibromyalgia, so why do our muscles hurt? Could something else in the muscle be generating pain signals and causing spinal cord hyper-reactivity?

There is indeed something abnormal in the muscles in fibromyalgia—we just have not been looking in the right part of the muscle. The problem lies not within the muscle cells themselves, but in the connective tissue wrapping around those cells. In the next chapter I present some new evidence that the pain signals may be coming from the fascia—the connective tissue that surrounds the muscle—and that this is the likely trigger for the spinal cord hyper-reactivity seen in fibromyalgia.

5

FASCIA IS THE SOURCE OF MUSCLE PAIN

"The scientist knows that in the history of ideas, magic always precedes science, that the intuition of phenomena anticipates their objective knowledge."

–Michel Gauqelin

In the last few chapters, we reviewed the well-known problems in both the pain and stress response in fibromyalgia. Now we venture into more uncharted territory and look at emerging research that the fascia (the connective tissue surrounding the muscle) causes the muscle pain in fibromyalgia. The idea of dysfunction in the fascia puts the pieces of the fibromyalgia puzzle together in a way that makes scientific sense.

Fascia and fibromyalgia
My personal experience of pain relief with therapy directed at the fascia led me to suspect that it was the source of pain in fibromyalgia. Through years of studying this topic, I have found evidence supporting the theory that the fascia may indeed be the trigger for the spinal cord hyper-reactivity in fibromyalgia.[1]

This is not actually a new idea. A physician proposed in 1904 that inflammation of "white fibrous tissue" around the muscles was the source of fibromyalgia pain, then called fibrositis or chronic rheumatism.[2] Later that year another physician studying muscle biopsies reported evidence of inflammation in the connective tissue of the muscle. Dr. Ralph Stockman found swelling and proliferation of cells in the connective tissue surrounding the fibromyalgia muscle and concluded, "The essential pathological changes in chronic rheumatism are confined to white fibrous tissue."[3]

However, he thought this inflammation was the result of the connective tissue being infected by a bacteria. When later studies did not show any evidence of infection or bacteria in the connective tissue, his findings were dismissed by the scientific community.

More recently another physician reported abnormalities in the connective tissue surrounding muscle cells in fibromyalgia. Dr. Essam Awad published a paper in 1973 describing his findings of increased cells and swelling in the connective tissue of muscles of fibromyalgia patients. He wrote that the abnormalities he saw in the biopsies indicated "the presence of a disorder primarily involving the connective tissue" of the muscles in fibromyalgia.[4]

Patients have told me this too, although not in these exact words. "It hurts on the outside of my muscles," one recently told me, and another said her muscles felt swollen. Patients have reported to me that their massage therapists tell them their fascia feels thick and excessively tight.

But if you were to ask your doctor about the fascia, they might not be able to tell you much because "medical books barely mention fascia and anatomical displays remove it."[5] This may explain why the role of fascia in causing fibromyalgia pain has been ignored up until recently. However, there are many researchers now studying the fascia. Their research, along with my own experience and that of my patients, has contributed to this theory.

Those studies that found no abnormalities in fibromyalgia muscles might have been just not looking at the right place within the muscle. It is important to remember that these studies were only looking at the muscle cells themselves and not at the connective tissue wrapping around the muscles. Two recent studies looking specifically at the fascia did find abnormalities that may finally explain why the muscles hurt in fibromyalgia.

What exactly is the fascia?

First we need to take a step back and describe the fascia, which is the connective tissue that surrounds and supports every muscle in the body, along with forming the tendons that insert into bone. This connective tissue also occurs alone in thick bands that give structural support to the body, like the plantar fascia at the bottom of the foot.

On my first day of gross anatomy class in medical school, after cutting into our cadaver I was shocked to see that every muscle was covered in a beautiful, iridescent, shiny white coating. This coating was wrapped around each muscle and was really strong and tough.

What I was seeing was the fascia, wrapping tightly around each muscle as a whole and binding the muscle cells together. It's a connective tissue sheath that surrounds every bundle of muscle fibers and even each individual muscle cell. Essentially each muscle is made up of thousands of long springs—the muscle cells—bound together into a tight bunch by multiple layers of connective tissue wrapping.

Imagine hundreds of long rubber bands (the muscle cells) each wrapped individually in tape (the fascia). Small bundles of these tape-covered rubber bands are grouped together and wrapped in more tape, and then all the small bundles are wrapped together with one large sheet of tape to create

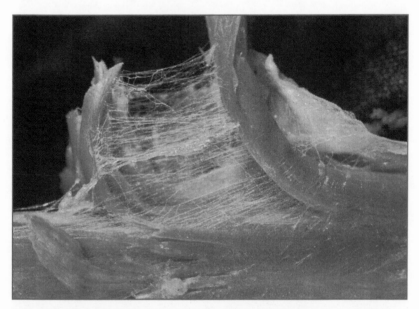

Figure 1: Dissection photograph of human fascia. (Photo by Ron Thompson.)

one large bundle. This creates a very strong, compact muscle working in unison, much stronger than if you just had a loose bunch of rubber bands.

The geometry of the fascia is fascinating. It is an intricate honeycomb of connective tissue, intimately linked with the muscle and continuous with the tendons. You probably have seen the outer layer of fascia before as the translucent covering you can peel away from a chicken breast. Figure 1 is a dissection photograph of human fascia. Figure 2 illustrates the organization of the three different layers of the fascia that are connected in a large web that merges into the tendon and bone.

The connective tissue around the muscle is highly sensitive to pain and actually has more nerve endings that transmit pain signals than the muscle cells themselves.[6-8] In fact, the fascia is about as sensitive to pain as our skin. Needles inserted into the thick outer layer of fascia surrounding the muscle hurt more than needles poked deep into the muscle tissue itself.[9]

Fascia is composed of cells suspended in a gel called the extracellular matrix, similar to shells embedded in the wax of a candle. There are some scattered immune cells, but most of the cells are fibroblasts that have long, spidery, finger-like projections. The fibroblast secretes all the components of the "goo" that surrounds them, and produces the tough fibers of collagen and stretchy fibers of elastin that are also suspended in the gel. The collagen fibers give the fascia its strength, and elastin fibers provide elasticity and stretch. This dense gel filled with cells and fibers forms a tough, protective coating around the muscles that has the unique ability to adapt and remodel in response to mechanical stress from wear and tear.

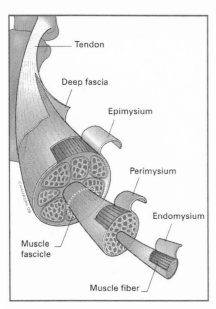

Figure 2: Three layers of the fascia

This massive connective tissue network surrounding the muscle transmits the forces generated from the contracting muscle fibers to the surrounding bones, allowing for movement to occur. The fascia is also the shock absorber of the muscle tissue and suffers the most damage from movement, much more so than the muscle cells themselves. As the glue holding the muscle fibers together, it is the part of the muscle most damaged with repeated motion or mechanical strain. The fascia serves as a supportive structure around the muscle cells and actually leads the way in repairing muscle damage after trauma.

The cells of the fascia direct the repair process of muscle by secreting more collagen, more "goo" and chemicals that attract immune cells to the area of damage. The muscles of mice that are forced to walk on a treadmill for prolonged periods show increased fibroblasts, collagen, and immune cells in the fascia during the 5–20 days it takes for the muscles to repair themselves.[10] Muscle biopsies of rats that have run downhill for 90 minutes show dramatically increased immune cells in the fascia, along with very active fibroblasts that are churning out collagen.[11] Interestingly, the muscle cells themselves show minimal immune system or repair activity. It is mostly in the surrounding connective tissue.[12, 13]

The fibroblasts in the fascia seem to direct muscle tissue repair. They respond to tissue damage and muscle strain by secreting extra collagen to provide more strength. They also secrete chemicals that draw immune cells to the area to help with tissue remodeling, and play a key role in the healing of wounds and creating of scar tissue.[14] In response to tissue injury, some fibroblasts are even able to contract in order to pull the edges of wounds together.[15]

The muscle tissue—and especially the surrounding fascia—is continually engaged in a process of damage and repair. Fibroblasts are continually repairing the collagen network in which they reside, similar to a spider repairing its web. When the rate of damage to the muscle is higher than the rate of repair, excessive collagen and scar tissue development can result. Rats whose muscles are repeatedly exercised without adequate recovery time develop excess collagen in the fascia of the over-exercised muscles.[16]

Muscles from frequent marathon runners show scarring and extra collagen between the muscle fibers.[17]

If you think back to the rubber band and tape analogy I used earlier, it makes sense that with repeated stretching the tape would start becoming frayed first, but the rubber bands themselves would remain undamaged. If the frayed tape is not adequately replaced, the small tears could turn into larger tears. Or if too much tape is used to repair the damage, the result would be a stiff and sticky mess.

In some situations, such as plantar fasciitis and tendinitis, the repair process is not able to keep up with the damage, resulting in chronic inflammation and pain. When tissues are under excessive strain or the repair process is inadequate, tissue repair and remodeling can become dysfunctional. A dysfunctional tissue healing response is seen in many conditions of chronic tissue strain such as tendinitis or repetitive stress injuries. Too much collagen, laid down in a haphazard pattern, can result in painful scarring, thickening, and adhesions of the fascia.

A good example of this is plantar fasciitis, a painful inflammation of the thick band of fascia on the bottom of the foot. Under a microscope, the fascia in patients with plantar fasciitis appears thickened, with excessive and disorganized collagen.[18, 19] Similar findings of abundant chaotic collagen are seen in biopsies of elbow tendinitis (tennis elbow).[20] Tendinitis is a repetitive stress injury in which the tendon tissue is not able to heal before it is damaged again by strain or stress.

The same type of tissue changes were observed in one study of chronic low back pain sufferers. Ultrasound assessment revealed approximately 25 percent thicker tissue in the fascia surrounding their low back muscles than in people without back pain.[21] A biopsy study of low back fascia found evidence suggestive of inflammation with degenerative changes in the collagen fibers and scarring.[22]

As you will see, similar changes in the fascia have been described in fibromyalgia, indicating that the balance of tissue damage and repair is abnormal. The most painful areas of the muscles in fibromyalgia, the tender points, occur in those locations that suffer the most strain and damage from daily muscle movement. The areas where muscles join tendons are particularly susceptible to injuries from wear and tear and many of the fibromyalgia tender points occur in those areas.

Anyone who has experienced the foot pain associated with plantar fasciitis knows how painful an inflammation of the fascia can be. A dysfunctional healing response of the fascia may result in pain and inflammation in muscles throughout the body, almost like a body-wide fasciitis. This process has already been described in smaller areas of fascia in conditions such as tendinitis, plantar fasciitis, and low back pain. In fibromyalgia, the fascia around all the muscles may be unable to repair itself adequately from even usual daily muscle activity, resulting in inflammation and pain.

The fascia in fibromyalgia

People with fibromyalgia often tell me their muscles feel "bruised" or similar to the muscle soreness normally experienced the day after intense or unusual exercise—only much worse. We used to think that lactic acid buildup in muscles is what caused this type of post-exercise soreness. Most experts have rejected this theory, because multiple studies have shown that by one-hour post exercise, lactic acid levels in the muscles are back to normal. The post-exercise muscle soreness is now thought to be due primarily to the chemicals released during the repair process in the muscle and connective tissue.

Muscle activities that tend to cause the most post-exertional muscle pain are eccentric exercises. Eccentric exercise refers to any type of muscle movement where a muscle has to lengthen at the same while it is tensed. Imagine you are holding a heavy box, and then set it down. As you do, your arm muscles are tensed to hold up the weight of the box, but you are also lengthening those tensed muscles as you place the box down. Other examples of eccentric exercise include running downhill, because your thigh muscles are tensed to keep you upright against gravity, but also lengthening as you take each step. Eccentric exercise transmits a great deal of force through the connective tissue of the muscle resulting in multiple micro-injures to the collagen in the fascia. As collagen strings rip apart, they release chemicals that attract immune cells to the area and trigger fibroblasts to start making more collagen to repair the damage.

Healthy muscles that are strained by over-exercise—especially eccentric exercise—consistently demonstrate increased collagen and immune cells in the fascia.[23-25] A few studies have found similar changes in the fascia of fibromyalgia patients, but without the intense exercise to explain the tissue damage. But consider that in fibromyalgia, the fascia is tightened under the direction of the fight-or-flight nervous system, so the muscles are constantly moving against tension. Essentially any movement in fibromyalgia becomes an eccentric, and damaging, exercise. Combine this with an inadequate tissue healing response related to lack of deep sleep and growth hormone, and you have the recipe for significant muscle pain.

Two recent studies using specialized staining techniques of fibromyalgia muscle biopsies have revealed excessive and disorganized collagen and increased release of immune cells and chemicals. These abnormalities suggest excessive tissue damage in the fascia in fibromyalgia. As we know from other similar conditions such as plantar fasciitis and tendinitis, this can result in tissue pain and soreness.

One study found an increase in collagen in the fascia of fibromyalgia patients. Comparing specially stained muscle biopsies, researchers described a "slight, but significant, increase in collagen surrounding the muscle cells of the fibromyalgia patients."[26] Another study also found increased levels of collagen, along with excessive immune cells and inflammatory chemicals in the connective tissue between fibromyalgia muscle cells.[27]

Specifically they noted elevated levels of N-carboxymethyllsine (CML), a marker of oxidative stress and tissue damage, in the fascia of fibromyalgia patients. Importantly, the increased staining for the markers of tissue damage was not inside the muscle cells but found mostly in the area between the muscle cells—the fascia. Along with high levels of tissue damage markers, they reported increased staining of three different types of collagen. The increased collagen and tissue damage markers occurred together, suggesting that the tissue damage was related to collagen.

They also found increased levels of macrophages (a type of white blood cell that is key in immune responses) and activated NF-kB in the fascia.

NF-kB is a protein that when activated plays an important role in the regulation of inflammation, and high levels of this protein are also seen in joints inflamed due to rheumatoid arthritis.[28] This protein is particularly important in the inflammatory and repair response of muscle tissue.[29] Taken together, these two studies suggest excessive tissue damage and ineffective repair of the fascia in fibromyalgia.

But what could cause these problems in the fascia in fibromyalgia?

Chronic activation of the fight-or-flight response may promote tension in the fascia of the muscles and lead to tissue damage. The fight-or-flight nervous system seems to stimulate the fascia to contract, which may be beneficial in emergencies but harmful when it is engaged chronically. Studies showing elevated pressures inside the muscles of fibromyalgia may reflect the tightening of the fascia in response to danger signals coming from the fight-or-flight nervous system. Muscles and fascia that are constantly tensed in fight-or-flight mode are more prone to injury and damage from even usual everyday activity. The lack of deep sleep and inadequate growth hormone leads to inadequate tissue healing response in the fascia.

Fascia is not just an inert covering wrapped around the muscle. The cells of the fascia are able to contract on their own, even without the muscle cells. This contractile ability may contribute to the incredible feats of strength humans can perform in emergencies. Temporarily, the fascia is able to stiffen or tense and give additional strength beyond what the muscle cells alone can usually produce. Consider again the muscle as a rubber band bundle wrapped in layers of tape. If you could suddenly stiffen or contract all the surrounding tape at once, the rubber band bundle would be able to provide enormous strength, at least temporarily.

Researchers believe that rapid contraction of the fascia is what creates the enormous extra strength that humans can produce in emergencies; for example, when a mother lifts a 2,000 lb. car to rescue her child, or fights off a much stronger male attacker.[30] These emergency situations are when the fight-or-flight response is most activated and is able to generate extreme muscle tension and strength.

People with fibromyalgia often tell me it feels like every fiber in their body is tensed, and I think this reflects tightening of the fascia in the fight-or-flight response. Fascia is like the armor of the body, tensing and contracting to protect us. I often notice my body feeling tense and coiled, as if ready to leap into action at any point. A patient described to me that her muscles always feel "all bunched up and tight."

Sometimes I wake up and feel as though my jaw, and entire body, have been clenched all night. One patient told me that she wakes up in the middle of the night, and her whole body and jaw are tensed up. This is clearly not a conscious tensing of the muscles, because it occurs even while sleeping and unconscious. This tension in the fascia is part of the automatic response to stress, and is not under conscious control.

Several studies have measured higher levels of tension in the fascial tissue in fibromyalgia. One found increased muscle electrical activity: "In terms of muscle relaxation, this suggests that fibromyalgia patients are not able to reach the normal baseline of healthy controls in rest."[31, 32] Other researchers inserted a pressure gauge needle and found increased pressure inside the fibromyalgia muscles compared to normal healthy controls.[33]

Fight-or-flight response and the fascia

New evidence indicates there may be direct nerve linkages from the fight-or-flight nervous system to the fascia. In order to have a rapid response to danger, there needs to be a direct connection between the fight-or-flight nervous system and the fascia. For a stress response action to be effective it has to be immediate, essentially a reflex, and would need direct nerve connections in order to do that.

Recent biopsy studies have shown that there are many fight-or-flight nerves running throughout the fascia. A professor of anatomy at the University of Freiburg describes a "direct connection of fascia with the autonomic nervous system."[34]

Fibroblasts (the major cells of the fascia) have specific receptors for the chemicals secreted by the fight-or-flight nervous system.[35] Fibroblasts respond directly to these chemicals by multiplying faster and increasing their secretion of collagen.[36] This indicates there may be direct communication between the cells of the stress response system and the cells of the fascia.

In the lab, fibroblasts contract most strongly in response to TGF-beta-1, a chemical that is secreted by immune cells when they are stimulated by fight-or-flight chemicals.[37] According to Dr. Robert Schleip, a leading fascia researcher, sympathetic nervous system activation causes increased fascial tightness. This relationship occurs in the opposite direction as well. Reducing fascial tone through stretching and manual therapy decreases fight-or-flight nervous system activation.[34]

Putting it all together

Fascial dysfunction and inflammation may be the cause of the widespread muscle pain in fibromyalgia. Excess tension in the fascia due to activation of fight-or-flight system may lead to excessive tissue damage, similar to over-exercised muscles. As you have seen, two different studies found increased collagen and inflammation in the fascia in fibromyalgia. In response to excess tension and tissue damage, fibroblasts secrete more collagen and immune chemicals in a continuous attempt to repair the damage. But in fibromyalgia there are two major factors inhibiting tissue repair: not having enough deep sleep or growth hormone.

The lack of deep sleep—a critical time for body tissue repair and remodeling—does not provide adequate repair time for the strained and damaged fascia. Growth hormone deficits further worsen the situation, since fibroblasts are dependent on this hormone for proper functioning. Fibroblasts have growth hormone receptors, and in response to this hormone secrete many important locally acting growth factors that regulate normal tissue healing.[38, 39] Research shows improved wound and tissue healing after administration of human growth hormone.[40, 41] Not enough growth hormone could lessen the ability of fibroblasts in the fascia to repair damage and worsen the inflammation.

Chronic fight-or-flight activation prevents deep sleep and impairs growth hormone release. It may also lead to excess tension of the fascia, poor tissue healing, and even fibrosis and adhesions. If the fascia is unable to repair the constant micro-trauma from everyday activities, this would produce a state of chronic inflammation as fibroblasts over-produce immune chemicals and collagen. This inflammation irritates nerve endings in the fascia, causing muscle pain and soreness. Constant pain signals coming from the fascia could overwhelm the spinal cord and induce a state of hyper-reactivity to pain or central sensitization.

Pathway To Central Sensitization In Fibromyalgia

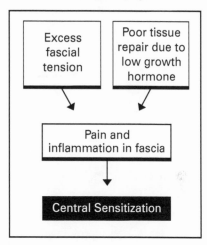

These are early results, and much more research needs to be done. But dysfunction in the fascia may fill in the gap in our understanding as to what actually hurts in fibromyalgia. This could enable us to focus treatments on the fascia to effectively reduce pain. If we were to reduce the pain signals coming from the fascia, we could decrease muscle pain and potentially reduce or eliminate the spinal cord hyper-reactivity. See Chapter 11 for more information on ways to treat fascial dysfunction.

CHAPTER RESOURCES

FASCIA: Clinical Applications for Health and Human Performance by Mark Lindsay

For current research information: www.fasciaresearch.com

6

CAUSES OF INFLAMMATION

Another result of the chain reaction starting with a stress response stuck in fight-or-flight mode is a body-wide, generalized inflammation. This low-grade inflammation results in feeling achy and flu-like, and contributes to fatigue and muscle pain.

Inflammation represents the immune system's response to tissue injury or foreign material (viruses, bacteria, etc.). There is evidence for overall mild activation of the immune system in fibromyalgia. Several studies have found high levels of cytokines, chemical messengers of the immune system, in fibromyalgia. This suggests the presence of an inflammatory response. Most doctors and researchers agree there is no severe and dramatic inflammation like that seen with bacterial infections or in diseases like rheumatoid arthritis. But a few well-designed studies show evidence for a more low-grade chronic inflammation in fibromyalgia. Some other studies have had conflicting results, however, and this is quite a controversial topic.

Certainly I can always tell when I am coming down with a flu or a cold, both situations when your body is flooded with inflammatory cytokines, because my usually low-grade fibromyalgia symptoms become suddenly and dramatically worse. Many of my patients also report a similar connection. This pattern, along with the results of several studies has confirmed my belief in the involvement of an immune response and inflammation in fibromyalgia.

One study documented higher blood levels of IL-6, a pro-inflammatory cytokine in fibromyalgia subjects, leading the authors to suggest "the possibility that inflammation and/or immune activity may contribute to symptoms in these patients."[1]

Another study found elevated inflammatory cytokines IL-10, IL-8, and TNF-alpha in fibromyalgia patients compared to controls, which the authors describe as a "chronic sub-inflammation."[2] A third study followed fibromyalgia patients and found that the higher levels of inflammatory cytokines persisted over six months.[3]

Sickness behavior

Any foreign invader into the body, such as a flu virus, is greeted by an armada of immune system cells that release chemicals to regulate the process of inflammation. Some of these chemical regulators promote inflammation, while others have anti-inflammatory effects. The inflammatory cytokines released during an immune response are what actually cause the fatigue and muscle aches experienced during an illness.

In healthy lab animals, injections of certain cytokines can cause what is called "sickness behavior"—lethargy and decreased social and reproductive behaviors. In humans, this is expressed as fatigue, poor appetite, muscle aches, and low energy.[4] Administration of inflammatory cytokines to healthy people results in fatigue, pain, depression, and decreased cognitive function.[5]

The observation of fibromyalgia-like symptoms in cancer patients treated with certain cytokines, and the similarities between the symptoms of sickness behavior and fibromyalgia, have lead to a great deal of research interest in this area over the past decade.

Inflammatory cytokines in the bloodstream also trigger a release of cytokines from glial cells in the central nervous system. These immune and support cells surround the neurons in the brain and spinal cord. The process of central sensitization has been linked to the activation of these cells. Systemic inflammation in the blood in fibromyalgia may be important in producing the central hypersensitivity to pain by triggering glial cell activation.[6]

What could cause generalized low-grade inflammation in fibromyalgia?

The inflammation in fibromyalgia comes from three different pathways that all start with the chronic activation of the fight-or-flight response.

First, as we learned in the last chapter, the fascia is in a constant state of inflammation as the body attempts to repair tissue damage. Second, sleep deprivation itself is known to result in elevated levels of immune cells and inflammatory chemicals such as cytokines.[7] Finally, there is another factor that we will learn about in this chapter; an immune response to foreign substances in the blood.

A stress response stuck in fight-or-flight mode can lead to poor sleep, but it also leads to poor digestion. The function of digestion is controlled by the autonomic, or "autopilot," nervous system. When the autopilot nervous system is in the fight-or-flight mode, blood and energy are diverted away from any non-essential activities, such as digestion, in order to allow you to have enough blood flow to escape from danger.

One of the most important functions of the digestive system is the regulation of what the intestines allow or reject for absorption into the blood stream. The dysfunction of the digestive system seen in fibromyalgia goes beyond just constipation and diarrhea, but also affects how and what nutrients are absorbed across the intestinal wall and enter the bloodstream.

How normal intestinal absorption works

After food is broken down into small particles in the stomach, the tiny pieces can be absorbed through the walls of the intestine into the bloodstream. The walls of the small intestine are very thin—only a single layer of cells. This single layer of cells has the very important job of allowing nutrient absorption across, while at the same time keeping out potentially harmful chemicals, bacteria, and viruses. Absorption of nutrient primarily occurs through the cells of the small intestine with special "doors" that open and shut to allow selected particles through and keep unwanted particles out.

Think of the doors on the intestine cell walls as being guarded by nightclub bouncers: For the most part they approve everything that goes past them, but a few very small things might sneak in through a side door, directly into the bloodstream. Part of the body's protection against these invaders is binding each intestinal cell closely to its neighbors so as to make these side doors very small.

Transport of Particles Across Intestinal Wall

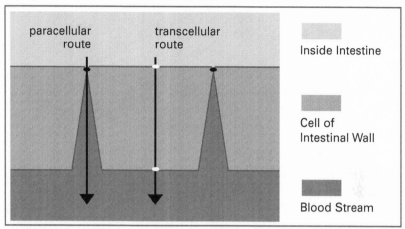

Particles can move through the intestinal cells (transcellular) or between the cells (paracellular) to get into the bloodstream

Each intestinal cell is tightly bound to its neighbors by "tight junctions," similar to the horizontal boards that connect individual fence posts to create a fence. While most of the nutrient absorption does occur across pores or "doors" through the cells themselves, some small substances can bypass the cells and sneak between the fence posts. Once a toxin or bacteria breaches that single layer of cells, they essentially have free access to the bloodstream.

A leaky gut

Normally, only a very small amount of particles can slip between these fence posts of the intestinal cells. But in certain situations, the posts can move further apart and the gaps between the cells can become bigger, allowing entrance of larger substances. This phenomenon is well known in the world of alternative medicine as the "leaky gut syndrome." As a consequence, some bacteria, incompletely digested proteins and fats, and other substances may enter the bloodstream and trigger an immune system response just as any foreign invader would. An intriguing recent study demonstrated that patients with fibromyalgia have "leakier" intestines than healthy subjects. In this study, fibromyalgia patients showed much higher absorption of a substance that normally should be too big too fit through the walls of the intestine, on average allowing nearly twice as many large particles through as control subjects.[8]

What could cause increased intestinal permeability in fibromyalgia? Emerging research demonstrates that intestines leak more during the fight-or-flight response. These changes seem to be caused by stress hormones (corticosteroids) secreted by the adrenal glands. When rats are subjected to prolonged stress, they show an increase in intestinal leakiness. But this does not occur in rats whose adrenal glands are removed so they cannot make stress hormones, indicating the importance of the stress response in regulating intestinal permeability.[9]

Just like in rats exposed to stress, prolonged activation of the stress response in fibromyalgia could lead to intestinal leakiness. Interestingly, even artificial stress hormones, like medications such as corticosteroids, can increase gut leakiness, as can NSAIDS (non-steroidal anti-inflammatories).[10] In fact, studies show that NSAID medications increase intestinal permeability within 12 hours.[11] This may explain why anti-inflammatory medications like steroids and NSAIDS have never shown any benefit in studies for in fibromyalgia; they may be making the inflammation worse by increasing leakiness of the intestines.

Immune system reaction to foreign substances in the bloodstream

These studies do provide tantalizing evidence that in fibromyalgia the gut barrier may allow unwelcome particles access to the bloodstream, but the reactions that these foreign particles might cause in the body is another source of controversy.

Theoretically, if foreign food or chemical substances from the gut are entering the bloodstream, they can provoke an immune response just like any bacteria or virus. This is technically considered an allergy because it is an immune reaction to a normally harmless substance. But this terminology can be confusing, because when most people refer to allergy they mean one specific type of immune reaction; the type of immediate immune reactions seen in hay fever or seasonal allergies.

However, there are also delayed allergic reactions that develop over a period of several hours or days. These are entirely different immune processes from those seen in rapid reactions, such as hay fever. But because delayed reactions are difficult to investigate and confirm, the concept of food or other substances causing delayed immune reactions is quite controversial and not well accepted by conventional Western medicine.

Immune response and physical symptoms as reactions to ingested substances have been explored in other illnesses as well. A small study found that 30 percent of patients studied with rheumatoid arthritis had symptoms of joint pain, stiffness, and swelling that were exacerbated by eating certain foods. One patient with rheumatoid arthritis who identified milk and dairy products as worsening her symptoms was studied in detail. This patient exhibited marked improvement in both joint swelling and pain while fasting. Four different "blinded" challenges with milk reproducibly caused symptoms, but placebo and other food had no ill effects. Symptoms peaked 24–48 hours after challenge and resolved over 1–3 days. Blood tests done on this patient found markedly increased antibodies to milk in her blood, and her immune cells exhibited sensitivity after exposure to milk in the lab.[12] This indicates that milk particles were actually entering her blood stream and triggering an immune reaction.

Another study found that when rheumatoid arthritis patients were given an allergenic food after 12 days of avoiding that particular food, there was a notable rise in the levels of joint pain and inflammatory cytokines in the blood.[13]

Allergic myalgia
In fact, the idea that delayed immune response to foods could cause physical symptoms is not actually a new one. As early as the 1840s, a French physician noted that diet could affect the development of painful muscle aches. In the 1950s, Dr. Theron Randolph, a pioneering physician in the field of food allergy, described a condition he called "allergic myalgia." He thought that for certain individuals, sensitivities or "allergies" to food and chemicals resulted in symptoms of muscle aching, pain, and fatigue.

In a paper in 1951, he described four different patients with food and chemical sensitivities that resulted in aching and painful, tight muscles.[14] One patient described it as "the feeling of having been severely pummeled the preceding night." When these patients avoided the offending substances, their symptoms improved.

It's amazing to me how much his description of allergic myalgia also perfectly describes fibromyalgia: "Complaints of patients with these symptoms vary from nagging sensations of pulling, drawing, tautness, and aching of the involved muscles to violent and sharply localized pain and cramping sensations, both with and in the absence of nodular areas of increases firmness and tenderness in the bellies or insertions of the involved muscles. The affected muscles commonly become more rigid during sleep so that chronic symptoms are apt to be accentuated on arising in the morning."

Dr. Randolph diagnosed and treated allergic myalgia by admitting patients to the hospital and having them fast for days, then gradually trying different foods one at a time to see if they provoked symptoms. As you can imagine, this was a very expensive and time-consuming process.

Testing for allergies

So how can we figure out what foods are causing an immune response? Theoretically, many different substances may be inappropriately getting into bloodstream through a leaky gut, but not all will cause an immune response. Each person's food sensitivities are going to be different, because each of our bodies has a unique set of antibodies. We all have thousands of different antibodies floating around in our bloodstream, waiting to meet the exact antigen (or invader) that fits it.

You can think of antibodies as the lock, and antigens as the key. If a key cannot find a lock that fits it, the immune system will not be triggered. What triggers one person to have an immune response might have no effect on someone else.

There are two well-established tests for allergies used in conventional Western medical practice: the skin-prick test and radioallergosorbent testing (RAST). Unfortunately, these detect only rapid immune responses, which are caused by excessive activation of one type of antigen, called IgE. These rapid immune response are hay fever type allergies, and cause hives, wheezing, or shock that may appear minutes after being exposed to a reacting food or chemical.

Delayed food sensitivities are not caused by IgE activation, so cannot be tested for by skin-prick or RAST testing.[15] One way to look for delayed immune responses is a food elimination/challenge trial like Dr. Randolph used in the 1950s. Suspected foods are eliminated from the diet for a period of 10–14 days, then reintroduced (the challenge) and symptoms are observed.

Unfortunately, delayed immune responses are quite difficult to detect using a food elimination/challenge trial. Let's say you have an immune response to milk, but after drinking it your reaction is that you get a headache three days later. That is going to make connecting your headache to milk much tougher. If you do get a headache three days after drinking milk, how do you know it is due to the milk, and not a tension headache? Or from a reaction to the eggs you ate the day before?

Another major problem with using this sort of testing is that often the immune reactions are subtle and hard to quantify. In my personal experience, I found that some foods made me feel much more fatigued, achy, or depressed, or they decreased my concentration. Sometimes these effects were so subtle I wouldn't notice them for a few days, until I realized days later as I started to improve, *Hey, I've been in a funk and really tired the past few days*. Often I would describe it as more of a general feeling of ill-being, rather than any specific symptom.

So you can see the need for a test that looks for delayed immune responses. The enzyme-linked immunosorbant assay/activated lymphocyte cytotoxicity test (ELISA/ACT) appears to be that test. It has not been widely adopted by conventional medicine, but is used quite frequently by naturopathic physicians. It was actually developed by a physician and measures certain immune cells (the lymphocytes) reactivity to various substances.

The lymphocytes from a patient's blood sample are placed in incubation chambers and are then exposed to 350 different food and chemical substances. The reactivity of the lymphocytes to each substance is then measured by looking for specific increases in size and shape that activated lymphocytes are known to undergo. A sample is considered to be moderate in reactivity if 25–50 percent of the lymphocytes showed activation, and strongly reactive if more than 50 percent showed activation. The hundreds of substances tested include foods and food additives, environmental toxins, common medications, and only include material small enough to theoretically fit through the gaps of a leaky human intestinal tract.

Delayed immune system reactions in fibromyalgia

In a study published in the *Journal of Musculoskeletal Pain*, 40 fibromyalgia patients had their blood tested with the ELISA/ACT to detect delayed immune system reactions in the blood. Every single one of the fibromyalgia patients tested positive for multiple food/environmental sensitivities. The most frequent reactive substance was the commercial flavorant monosodium glutamate (MSG), followed by Candida albicans, caffeine, food coloring, chocolate, shrimp, and dairy products.

After the testing, some of the fibromyalgia patients continued their usual diet and lifestyle (the control group) and some made dietary changes to avoid the reactive substances (the treatment group) for six months. At both three and six months, the treatment group felt substantially better, with less pain and depression and more energy compared to pre-treatment.

In contrast, the control group that continued their usual diet reported increased levels of pain and depression, and similar levels of stiffness and energy as compared to the beginning of the study. Of course, the placebo effect cannot be excluded as a factor in this study, because each group obviously knew if they were in the dietary change group or not.

This study also did not look at ELISA/ACT results in healthy patients, only in subjects with fibromyalgia. However, according to the author of the study, previous work in their laboratory indicates that healthy normal subjects show only rare immune system reactions, the most common being to cow's milk and corn.[16]

Other studies have also shown improvement in fibromyalgia symptoms during periods of fasting or very limited diets (such as raw food or vegan), with worsening of symptoms once regular diet resumed.[17-19] I suspect that any benefit from fasting or eating a vegan diet is due to effectively eliminating most common allergens from the diet, rather than to any effect of the diet itself.

Pathways to inflammation

As we have learned, a leaky gut that allows unwelcome particles into the bloodstream is one result of the constant activation of the fight-or-flight nervous system in fibromyalgia. The immune response from food sensitivities may contribute to elevated levels of inflammatory chemicals in the blood and overall flu-like exhaustion and achiness.

Of course, it is overly simplistic to attribute *all* of the symptoms of fibromyalgia to food sensitivities. This is just the one of the end results from chronic fight-or-flight nervous system activation, but it is one of the easiest to treat in my experience, and is important to address. You will learn how to address this problem in Chapter 8.

CHAPTER RESOURCES

www.elisaact.com for blood allergy testing information

Food Allergy: Adverse Reactions to Foods and Food Additives edited by Dean Metcalfe, Hugh Sampson and Ronald Simon

An Alternative Approach to Allergies: The New Field of Clinical Ecology Unravels the Environmental Causes of Mental and Physical Ills by Theron G. Randolph

PART II

TREATING EACH STEP
IN THE CHAIN REACTION

7

A GUIDE TO GETTING BETTER

A patient told me recently that she felt like all she needed to get better from fibromyalgia was "some deep sleep and to unclench my body." And in essence, she's right. The lack of deep sleep is fundamental in causing the fatigue and pain of fibromyalgia. But there are ways to improve your sleep.

The muscles and fascia of the body are clenched in fibromyalgia in constant preparation for fight or flight. Myofascial release and other techniques can help the body unclench and reduce the stress response activation. Using gentle exercise as medicine stimulates growth hormone release and encourages deep sleep. With the right warm up, exercise doesn't have to hurt—and can really help. And changing your diet to avoid substances that cause an immune reaction reduces the achy and flu-like feelings of fibromyalgia.

Medical science has not yet figured out how turn off the switch of the stress response that gets stuck in the "on" position in fibromyalgia. When we do that, we will have found a cure. But right now there are some very effective treatments that address the end-results caused by the abnormal stress response.

As we reviewed in previous chapters, when the brain is stuck in the fight-or-flight mode it starts a chain reaction that leads to muscle pain, poor deep sleep, and fatigue. Treating the end results of this chain reaction, while not a cure, can result in significant improvement in fibromyalgia symptoms.

In Part I, you learned what goes wrong in fibromyalgia, and read about my personal journey to find effective treatments. It is not clear yet how to turn off or reverse the switch in the hypothalamus that is stuck in the fight-or-flight position. In the meantime, there are ways to improve deep sleep, reduce immune response to allergens, and reduce fascial tension and pain. These changes substantially improve symptoms.

Part II is a guide to these treatments. I have tried to make it as practical and useful as possible. Each treatment that I write about in the following chapters was helpful for me, and for the most part you could start them all at the same time, but I do not suggest this approach. First, I don't want you to get overwhelmed, as I remember feeling in my search for things that helped me. Second, I think it is really important to start with the ELISA/ACT testing, and to start avoiding those substances that cause your immune system to react. By doing that first, I was able to reduce the fatigue and body aches to the point that I had the energy and motivation to work on some of the other treatments, such as exercise and bodywork.

I highly recommend that you work with a medical practitioner to individualize your treatment to fit your specific needs. What worked for me might not work for everyone—the human body is more complex than that. But hopefully this book, along with your doctor, can be a guide towards finding the most effective treatment plan for you.

You can do this in any order or way that feels right. There may be other treatments you find that are helpful too. But based on my own experience, I would suggest this order:

1. Get diet/allergy testing and make appropriate changes.

2. Begin gentle exercise program, emphasizing the warm up.

3. Improve sleep habits, consider sleep medication to increase deep sleep.

4. Get bodywork focused on the fascia.

The next section, Part III, reviews other treatments for fibromyalgia, including supplements, alternative therapies, and prescription medications. In particular, I address which therapies are backed by research evidence so that you can make informed treatment decisions. I also include my own experiences with various treatments, along with those of my patients.

What does getting better mean for me?

Most days I don't even really feel like I have fibromyalgia anymore. In fact, I might not even technically meet the diagnostic criteria anymore, since I no longer have widespread muscle pain. I can still feel my fight-or-flight nervous system running the show. The baseline level of tension in my muscles and fascia is high. I have to remind myself frequently to take deep breaths, and consciously work on relaxing and forcing my body to switch into the rest-and-digest mode.

But the all-over body ache and flu-like feeling is gone. For the most part, I am pain-free, but if I use any one muscle in repetitive motion for too long (like twisting a screwdriver repeatedly), I will get painful in that local area. There is muscle tenderness if someone presses really hard, but generally my muscles don't hurt.

The more myofascial release therapy I get, the better I feel. The more gentle, regular exercise I do, the better I feel. I still wake up some mornings and feel like I've been clenching my jaw all night and have occasional flares of TMJ pain, which calm down after a few sessions of myofascial release (see Chapter 11 for more information about this type of therapy). I no longer have that prolonged stiffness and achiness in the morning that feels like all my muscles have hardened into rocks. When it does happen now it's localized to my jaw area.

My fatigue improved with Xyrem, a medication that induces deep sleep but is not currently FDA-approved for use in fibromyalgia. Even without this medication, my sleep is better than it used to be, and I don't wake up feeling as exhausted anymore. Read more about this medication in Chapter 10.

When you are tired and haven't had a night of deep sleep in years, it can be overwhelming to even think about doing any of these treatments. But you have the strength to do it—after all you have the strength to live with fibromyalgia every day. Empower yourself with knowledge and then take action.

My deepest hope is that my struggle and experiences over the past 10 years can help you feel better, too. My suggestions for your healing are only suggestions, and I definitely recommend you consult with your own physician or health care professional before starting any medication or exercise program.

8

PRACTICAL DIET ADVICE FOR FIBROMYALGIA

As you learned in Chapter 6, one result of stress response activation is increased leakiness of the intestines. This allows some unwelcome food particles access to the bloodstream. Chronic intestinal leakiness can lead to continual immune response to certain substances. This immune response can be experienced as achiness, fatigue, and a flu-like feeling.

People with fibromyalgia often tell me that their symptoms get worse after eating certain foods, but what bothers one person might be fine for another. As discussed in previous chapters, it can be difficult to figure this out just based on watching for patterns.

Most standard allergy tests don't test for this type of immune response to food or other substances. One particular test that does is the enzyme-linked immunosorbent assay/advanced cell test (ELISA/ ACT), which measures the reactivity of immune cells when exposed to different substances. It tells us how much certain white blood cells called lymphocytes respond to different common substances. The substances tested are only those that are small enough to fit through the gaps in a leaky intestinal tract and come into direct contact with white blood cells. They include foods, additives, preservatives, environmental chemicals, and medications.

Avoiding substances to which I was sensitive based on the ELISA/ACT blood test was the first treatment that substantially helped my fibromyalgia symptoms. I recommend this as a good place to start for patients for a few reasons. First, it is relatively easy to do. Second, avoiding these substances can help you to have the energy to devote to other effective treatments like bodywork and exercise.

Unfortunately, we do not yet have a way to turn off the fight-or-flight response or to stop the leakiness of the gut induced by the stress response. But determining which substances are generating an immune response, and then limiting exposure to them, can reduce symptoms. After a period of avoiding offending substances, the immune system can calm down over time to allow some to be tolerated again. Eating a varied diet can also reduce the development of food sensitivities.

How does the ELISA/ACT blood test work?

After avoiding anti-inflammatory medications for four days, and fasting overnight your blood is drawn and sent to the ELISA/ACT lab for analysis. This specialized test is done at only one laboratory in the country. The white blood cells called lymphocytes are separated from the rest of the blood, and then combined with more than 150 different substances. The response of your cells when combined with each substance is monitored over a few days and noted as non-reactive, moderately reactive, or strongly reactive. The more reactive your lymphocytes are to the substance, the more sensitive you are to it.

This type of testing is quite specialized, and costs around $300. On the ELISA/ACT website, you can find a health care provider that offers this type of testing. I will caution you that this website seems to claim that this testing is the solution to almost every health problem you can imagine, and I certainly do not think that is the case. However, in the specific case of fibromyalgia, there some supporting evidence to justify this type of testing.

When you get your test results back, they send along a very detailed nutrition booklet with multiple supplement and detoxification suggestions. Frankly, I found these overwhelming. I recommend just focusing on avoiding the substances to which you test positive.

There are two versions of the test, a basic version that tests around 150 substances, and a more comprehensive test that covers 300 substances. The basic version is adequate as long as you also switch to filtered water and use HEPA air filters to reduce your overall exposure to chemicals and molds as much as possible.

My experience with ELISA/ACT blood testing

My test results indicated that I had strong sensitivities to chicken, dairy, xanthan gum, carrots, watermelon, and blueberries. I also was moderately sensitive to a pesticide called methoxychlor and a few types of mold. I wondered if I was ever going to be able to eat chicken or butter again (*sob*).

My naturopath spent an hour with me reviewing the results and describing how to avoid or reduce my exposure to these substances. With the foods and additives, it was relatively straightforward: Don't eat them. She gave me some suggestions for butter substitutes. She also suggested I get a really good water filter, to decrease my exposure to pesticides such as methoxyxhlor which are common in city drinking water. Unfortunately, the common pitcher-style water filters don't actually filter very well. A good source for effective water filters is listed at the end of this chapter.

She suggested a high efficiency particulate air (HEPA) filter in the bedroom and living room to reduce the molds and other airborne particles in the air I was breathing at home. This type of filter can remove up to 99.7 percent of particles in the air, even very small particles such as pollen, dander, or mold spores.

So I bought water and HEPA filters, and avoided the foods and additives religiously. After about two weeks, I started to feel better with less body ache, flu-like feelings, and fatigue. I felt so much better when avoiding these substances that I continued to avoid them for about 18 months, much longer than is probably required

Many people asked me how I was able to stick to this regimen, since I had to avoid some of my favorite foods such as ice cream and butter. But actually, I felt so much better after I started that it wasn't really hard at all. "If every time you ate ice cream it made you feel like it makes me feel, you would have no problem avoiding it," I remember telling people.

After that, I began slowly re-introducing foods one at a time, and pretty much tolerated everything with no ill effects, although large amounts of dairy still produced a negative reaction. These days I continue to use a water filter and a HEPA filter, and just try to eat a varied diet.

Are these lifelong allergies?

Do you have to avoid these substances forever if you are "allergic" to them? Not necessarily. It is recommended that after getting the ELISA/ACT test results you avoid the offending items for three to six months, depending on the severity of the lymphocyte reaction. Then slowly reintroduce these substances one at a time after the avoidance period. It is suggested to retest within a year to identify any new sensitivities and to evaluate progress, although I was feeling so much better at that point I did not actually get a re-test.

These are not true "allergies" or intolerances. Rather they are substances that happen to be small enough to get through the gaps in your intestinal wall and that also happen to be activating an immune response. Sometimes giving the body a break from exposure to a substance allows your immune system to "forget" its sensitivity. A period of avoiding these substances may reduce sensitivity to them, and they can then be tolerated again in small quantities.

We tend to develop sensitivities to those things that we are exposed to the most frequently. I was responsive to chicken and dairy because I ate them in one form or another almost every day. One way to reduce potential sensitivities to food is to eat a varied diet. Don't eat the same things every day to avoid overdosing your system on any one food or food group. We all tend to get in ruts and eat the same foods every day, particularly when fatigue leaves little energy for food preparation.

In medical school I ate a protein bar for breakfast every day for months at a time, and had chicken breasts for dinner 3–4 times a week. In fact, Dr. Theron Randolph, a pioneering food allergy physician, recommended what he called the Rotary Diversified Diet, which involves eating one type of food no more than every four days, in addition to having a very diverse diet of non-processed foods. This means if you have wheat bread on Monday, you don't eat another wheat product such as pasta or cereal until Friday.

Certainly, this type of diet could be difficult to follow (unless you have a personal chef), but eating as varied a diet as possible will help reduce the development of food sensitivities.

Irritable bowel and bladder symptoms

The common symptoms of irritable bowel syndrome (IBS) may also improve when avoiding substances that are activating an immune response. Many people with fibromyalgia describe irregular bowel habits, and about 70 percent have enough symptoms to be diagnosed with irritable bowel syndrome.[1] This condition is characterized by abdominal pain, bloating, constipation, diarrhea, and nausea. It is very common to have alternating bouts of constipation and diarrhea.

Urinary symptoms, including bladder discomfort, urgency, and frequency of urination, are also associated with fibromyalgia. Some people have such severe bladder issues that they are diagnosed with interstitial cystitis, which is characterized by constant pressure and pain in the bladder area or lower pelvis along with urgency or frequency of urination.

The frequency of bowel and bladder irritability in fibromyalgia is explained by the fact that the functions of both are run by the autonomic or "autopilot" nervous system. The functions of digestion and elimination are mostly managed by the parasympathetic or "rest-and-digest" half of the of the autopilot nervous system. In fibromyalgia, where the balance in the autonomic nervous system is skewed so that fight-or-flight is dominant, the digestion and elimination functions get neglected. What you see is a digestive and urinary system that works haphazardly, in fits and starts, like a car with a transmission problem.

Bowel and bladder irritability can be very tricky symptoms to manage, and we don't have any great solutions yet. For patients with interstitial cystitis, I recommend seeing a urologist, as there are some very specific bladder injections that can be helpful in reducing bladder pain. Also a recent study showed myofascial release therapy reduced symptoms of interstitial cystitis.[2]

As far as my bowel symptoms, they did seem to improve after making dietary changes in response to the allergy testing. Another way to improve bowel function is to make sure the bacterial habitat in your intestines is as healthy as possible.

Overgrowth of yeast and bacteria in the gut

Normally, the bacteria and fungus that live in the human digestive tract only exist in the large intestine. However, when things get out of balance in the gut, a few things can happen. Bacteria normally only found in the large intestine can migrate up to the small intestine and take up residence there. This is called small intestinal bacterial overgrowth (SIBO). Having bacteria and fungus in the small intestine, where they should not normally reside, is thought to negatively affect the functioning of the small bowel and can lead to diarrhea, bloating, and gas. This appears to be very common in fibromyalgia. One study found that 100 percent of fibromyalgia subjects showed evidence of SIBO, as compared to only 20 percent of healthy subjects.[3]

There seems to be a link between small intestine bacterial overgrowth and irritable bowel symptoms of gas, bloating, diarrhea, and constipation.[3] In my experience, taking an acidophilus (healthy bacteria that is found in yogurt) supplement every day and reducing sugar intake seems to decrease irritable bowel symptoms.

The delicate balance between fungus and bacteria in the intestine can also be altered, leading to an overgrowth of fungus. One type of fungus, a yeast called Candida albicans, is of special concern. Any time we take antibiotics, it reduces the bacteria in our intestines and can lead to excessive growth of this yeast. Taking steroids and eating high sugar diets can also cause yeast to multiply out of control.

The problems that yeast overgrowth can cause are detailed beautifully in *The Yeast Connection Handbook,* by Dr. William Crook. An imbalance in yeast/bacteria levels can interfere with the proper functioning of the bowels. Yeast, in large quantities, can also be highly allergenic and cause the immune system to react to the yeast as a foreign invader. Many alternative health providers feel that yeast overgrowth can be responsible for a wide range of symptoms including fatigue, joint pain, and depression.

Candida albicans is a highly allergenic substance. In people with fibromyalgia, it was the second most common substance that elicited an immune response in one study using the ELISA/ACT test.[4] Because this yeast lives normally in your gut, it is impossible to avoid completely, but a diet that avoids sugars and minimizes carbohydrates can reduce the yeast overgrowth. Yeast in our gut, just like that used to make bread and beer, really like to eat sugar. Reducing sugar in your diet will slow yeast growth and some will die off. Other times, a course of antifungal medications or herbs might be needed, and many naturopaths treat this condition very well in my experience.

Final thoughts on food

You already know how to make your diet healthier: Increase fiber, fruit and vegetable consumption, and eat as much organic food as you can. Look into ordering groceries online and having them delivered. Buy prepared veggies and salads from the deli section at your local health food store, or prepare them yourself if you have the time. Minimize processed foods, particularly those with the food additives MSG and aspartame. If you recall, MSG was the number one substance that fibromyalgia sufferers were sensitive to in the study using ELISA/ACT testing (See Chapter 6 to read more about this study).

What has helped motivate me to eat better foods is the thought that at the level of the smallest particles, the food you eat will actually become part of your body. Although our body appears solid, it actually is in constant exchange with the outside world. The actual atoms, or very small particles, that make up your tissues quite literally come from the food you eat, the water you drink, and the air you breathe.

The atoms that make up the human body are like bricks that are built into intricate structures. While the structures—like the bones, muscles, and skin—keep their shape steady, over time the bricks themselves are constantly being replaced. Imagine a brick building in which every day one brick is replaced by a new one. Eventually, the building would look the same but entire structure would be made of new bricks. In fact, it is estimated that in one year, 98 percent of the atoms of the human body will be replaced.

So if you eat poor quality food, you get poor quality bricks in your tissues. If you eat high quality food, you get high quality bricks. Puts the old saying "You are what you eat" in a whole new perspective.

CHAPTER RESOURCES

For good water filters: www.multipure.com

You can learn more about the ELISA/ACT test, and find a healthcare practitioner in your area that utilizes this test at www.elisaact.com, or call 800-553-5472.

The Yeast Connection Handbook by William G. Crook

Fibromyalgia: My Journey to Wellness by Claire Musickant. Details one woman's experience with ELISA/ACT testing.

9

SOLVING THE
EXERCISE DILEMMA

More than 75 studies to date have shown the benefits of exercise in fibro-myalgia.[1] The challenge is that when you hurt all over and are exhausted, the last thing on earth you want to do is exercise. Trust me, I know!

When I was diagnosed with fibromyalgia, everything I read told me that regular exercise was important, but it seemed every time I exercised I felt worse afterwards. I often felt like I had strained a muscle, and my muscles felt more achy and tight after exercise.

I also frequently injured myself while exercising. I pulled a muscle in my neck while swimming and I remember wondering how I managed to injure myself with such a gentle exercise? Soon after starting a regular walking pro-gram, I developed heel pain and plantar fasciitis. I usually felt wiped out for days after exercising. So, even though I knew it was supposed to be helpful, I tended to avoid exercise until I learned how to do it without injuring myself.

Muscles in fibromyalgia are easily injured and less able to heal because of a lack of deep sleep, a lack of growth hormone, and tightness of the fascia. So you have to exercise with that in mind. That is why you need to warm up correctly, exercise gently, and ensure enough rest and recovery time between sessions. You can also improve your muscle recovery and exercise tolerance by improving your deep sleep, and using therapies like myofascial release to reduce scar tissue in the fascia.

So if muscles are prone to injury in fibromyalgia, why on earth should you exercise? If done right, exercise can help you to have less pain and fatigue. We know that exercise is a trigger for release of growth hormone, something the fascia in fibromyalgia is very hungry for.

Exercise also promotes deep sleep. Athletes have been noted to spend more time in deep sleep after exerting significant physical effort during the day.[2] Finally, exercise causes the release of endorphins, the body's natural painkillers.

What is a good warm up?

Ben Benjamin, the sports medicine and massage expert who helped me with a repetitive stress injury in my arms, also taught me how to exercise correctly. He has a Ph.D. in sports medicine and is the author of multiple books on the subject.

Ben emphasized the importance of exercise, but explained that when you have chronic muscle tension as in fibromyalgia, you have to be extra careful about warming up. I remember assuring him that I did a good warm up, describing my routine of doing some stretches and then getting on the stationary bike and pedaling slowly for five minutes before starting at a faster pace.

I thought his eyes were going to burst out of his head. "No, that is not a warm up!" he exclaimed. "A warm up starts out lying on the floor, and you do it before you do any exercise. And stretching definitely does not equal warming up." He told me that everyone should warm up before exercising to decrease their risk of injuring themselves because warm, relaxed muscles are much less likely to get hurt than cold, tight ones.

He described the warm up plan he had developed in his many years of working with people with sports injuries. You begin by lying on your back, wiggling your toes; then do ankle circles, and progressively work up the body. The whole process takes about 15 minutes. He gave me a copy of his book, *Exercise without Injury*, which included a whole chapter on warming up.

The next time I went to the gym, I dutifully tucked his book into my bag, and did exactly as he suggested. The whole exercise experience was much less painful; afterwards I felt tired but relaxed instead of achy and tight.

Why had nobody told me this before? I knew I had found a key component to effective and helpful exercise in fibromyalgia. I now use his routine before any type of exercise, and it has made a huge difference for me, both how much exercise I can tolerate and in how I feel afterward. I actually started playing soccer again, which I had not done since high school.

The warm up is particularly important in fibromyalgia. Because of the excess fascial tension due to the overactive stress response, it takes longer to get "the juices" flowing and the tissues loose and warm.

Over the years, I have gradually come up with my own adaptation of Ben's warm up program that I use everyday, and with his kind permission I will share my version of his warm up plan with you. You can spend as long as you like in each stage of the warm up, but don't focus too much on any one body part, and make sure you are frequently alternating your motions so as to not cause any strain. If any exercise doesn't feel right, you can slow it down, or modify it in any way that feels better to you.

How to do a good warm up

The first step is to literally get your body temperature up by sitting in a heated room, taking a hot shower or bath, or lying under a blanket. Warmth is essential to an effective warm up because muscles are looser when your temperature is slightly elevated. The point is to get your juices flowing, which in fibromyalgia might take a little extra time and care. See pages 73 to 77 for illustrations of these movements.

- On a yoga mat or carpet, lay on your back with hands at your side and feet shoulder width apart and legs flat on the ground.

- Take a few slow deep breaths.

- **Toe Curl:** Slowly curl and extend your toes a few times on both feet. (See figure 1.)

- **Ankle flex and circle:** Now bend your knees toward your chest and place your hands on your knees. Point and flex your feet slowly a few times, continually but gently move your ankles through their full range of motion up and down. Rest a few seconds, then gently circle your ankles through their full range of motion. You can do both ankles at once, or one at a time for this exercise. (See figure 2.)

- **Foot shake:** In the same position with knees toward your chest, shake your feet up and down for about 20–30 seconds, allowing your ankles to flop and your legs to be loose like jelly. If it is more comfortable place your hands under your low back to provide extra support in this position. (See figures 3 and 4.)

- **Basic position:** Put your feet back on the floor, with your knees bent. We'll call this the basic position. (See figure 5.)

- **Knee to chest:** From the basic position, bring one knee toward your chest and then return your leg to the basic position. Bring the other leg toward your chest, and then back to basic position. Alternate legs and do this about 4–5 times on each side. (See figure 6.)

- **Thigh squeeze:** Again raise your knees to your chest. This time slowly move your knees apart to the side, and then together again in the center. Do this in very small motions. You may be just moving a few inches either way, but you can gradually increase that as it feels comfortable. (See figure 7.)

- **Chest-extend-chest-replace:** From basic position, bring one leg toward your chest, and then straighten that leg so that it is held a few inches above the ground. Bend your leg back toward your chest, and then place it on the floor. So the pattern is chest-extend-chest-replace. Do this on both legs 4–5 times each. (See figure 8 and 9.)

- **Chest-extend-lift-replace:** From basic position, bring one leg toward your chest, then straighten your leg so that it is held a few inches above the ground, then lift that straightened leg towards the ceiling in the air, then bend your leg and return to basic position. The pattern is chest-extend-lift-replace. Do this 3–4 times with each leg. (See figure 10.)

- **Air bicycle:** Still lying on your back, bring your knees to your chest so that your knees and feet are both above your abdomen. Place your hands underneath your buttocks to stabilize your pelvis, and then make gentle circling motions with your legs, as if you were riding a bicycle. Try to have your feet over your chest, not your pelvis, to reduce strain on your back. Do this for 10 seconds, then rest, then repeat for another 10 seconds. (See figure 11.)

- **Shoulder roll:** Stand up with feet shoulder-width apart. With arms hanging loosely at your sides, do some gentle shoulder rolls forward and backward.

You are finished with the basic warm up. Now you can do a few key stretches and then you are ready to exercise. The stretches that I personally find most helpful are described below; you might have other areas that you like to stretch before you exercise. However, leave the majority of your stretching until after you complete your exercise, when it really benefits your muscles the most. And don't spend more than one or two minutes stretching after the warm up, or you will start to cool down before you even get started with exercise.

The calf stretch: Facing a wall, with both your feet 2–3 feet away from it, lean your forearms on the wall, resting your forehead on the back of your hands. Now bend one knee and bring that knee forward towards the wall. Keep your other leg straight with the heel down. Do this stretch for 20–30 seconds, then switch to the other calf. (See figure 12.)

This stretch is really important because it can reduce some of the pressure of the plantar fascia in the base of the foot. I struggled on and off with heel and foot pain from plantar fasciitis until I learned this stretch from a foot doctor. I do this at least once a day, and always before and after I exercise.

The thigh/ankle stretch: Lying on the floor on your back, lift one leg straight in the air and hold your leg around the thigh. Allow this to stretch the back of your thigh for 20–30 seconds, then point and flex your ankle a few times. Start making very slow circles with your ankle, much slower than those you did while warming up. Allow your ankle to stay in each position for a few seconds as it moves around the circle.

The thigh/shin stretch: Bending forward at the waist, straighten one leg and put the heel of that foot on the ground. Bend the other leg slightly at the knee, and support your arms on the thigh of the bent leg. It is important to keep your back as straight as possible during this stretch. Do this for about 10 seconds on each leg. (See figure 13.)

Now that you are warmed up, how should you exercise?

The other important lesson I have learned about exercise in fibromyalgia is to build up the length of exercise sessions gradually, not to push myself too hard, and to listen to my body when it says *Stop!*

I tell patients to exercise like you are a stubborn 80 year-old grandmother: gently but persistently. I tend to recommend a very low impact exercise such as walking or using an elliptical machine or recumbent exercise bike. Exercising in warm water therapy pools—at a temperature of 88–92° F, roughly the temperature of a lukewarm bath—has been shown to be very well-tolerated in fibromyalgia.[3] Exercising in warm water may provide additional benefits, as the warmth can help reduce muscle pain, spasm, or stiffness.

And I recommend starting out with 5–10 minutes exercise sessions on the lowest setting of the exercise machine or slow walking. Often people with fibromyalgia (myself included) start an exercise program by trying to do the customary 20–30 minutes sessions recommended for weight loss and cardiovascular health, but suffer so much in the days following that they give up on exercise.

A patient told me that when she went into a warm-water therapy pool, she always felt wiped out for three days afterward, so she stopped going. When I asked her how long she stayed in the pool, her answer was, "Ninety minutes, because it felt so good." That is a guaranteed recipe for disaster in a fibromyalgia exercise program.

My personal fibromyalgia exercise routine in the beginning was a 15 minute warm up, five minutes on the elliptical machine, 10 minutes

Fig. 1 – Toe curl

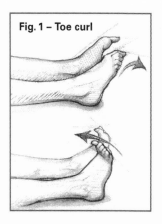

Fig. 2 – Ankle flex and circle

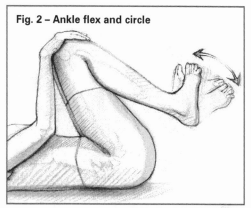

Fig. 3 – Foot shake

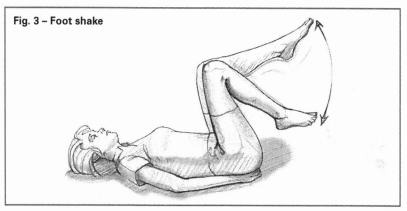

Fig. 4 – Low back support

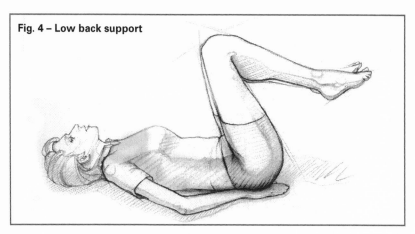

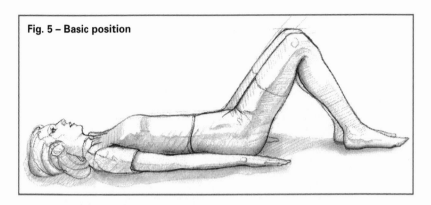

Fig. 5 – Basic position

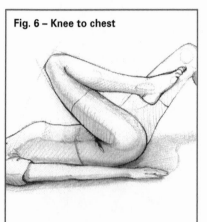

Fig. 6 – Knee to chest

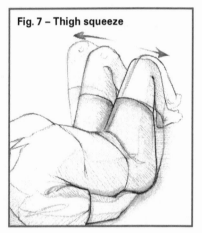

Fig. 7 – Thigh squeeze

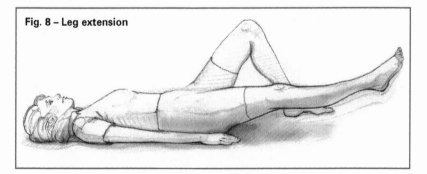

Fig. 8 – Leg extension

Fig. 9 – Chest-extend-chest-replace

A. Knee to chest

B. Leg extension

C. Knee to chest

D. Basic position

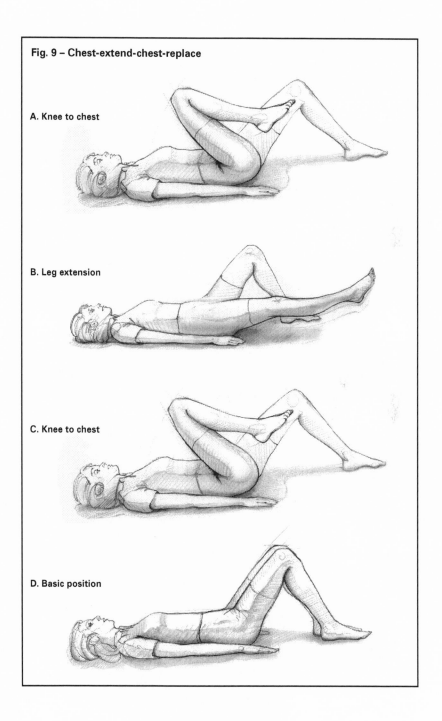

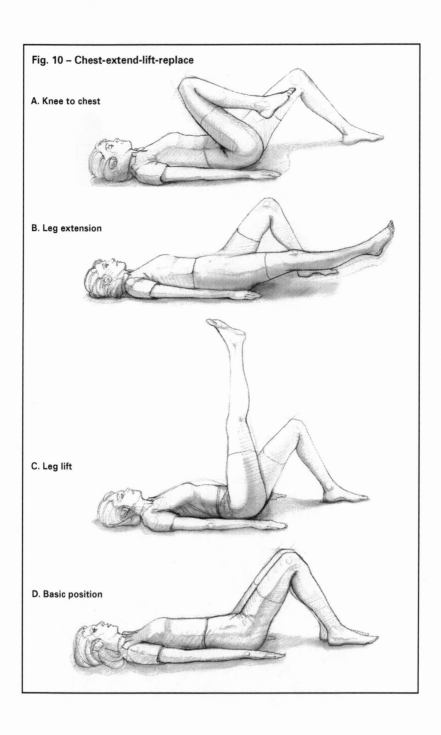

Fig. 10 – Chest-extend-lift-replace

A. Knee to chest

B. Leg extension

C. Leg lift

D. Basic position

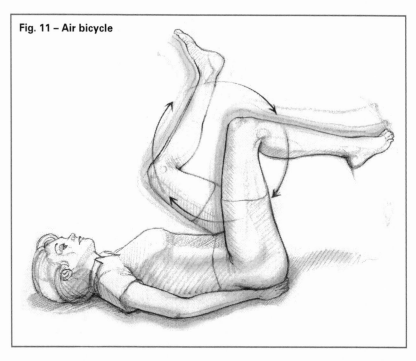

Fig. 11 – Air bicycle

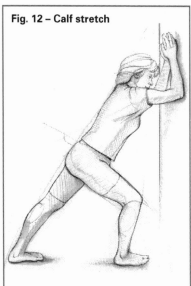

Fig. 12 – Calf stretch

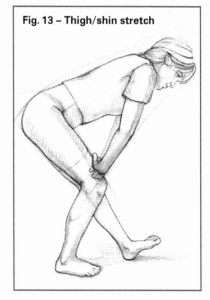

Fig. 13 – Thigh/shin stretch

of stretching, and that's it. I have gradually worked my way up to doing 15–20 minute elliptical sessions over a few years.

Even with that small amount of gentle exercise, I have found it works best in fibromyalgia to exercise every three days, to give your body adequate recovery and repair time. As you read in previous chapters, the repair process of muscle in fibromyalgia is slower. This stalled healing process is due to a number of different causes, including inadequate deep sleep and growth hormone, but it means that your body takes a little more time to recover. It is crucial to give yourself that time before going at it again.

Balance and exercise

It is also important to be aware of balance and low blood pressure issues when using exercise as medicine for fibromyalgia. About half of people with fibromyalgia report balance problems, which can range from mild to severe. Balance studies find that fibromyalgia sufferers have a hard time maintaining balance when asked to do a secondary cognitive task—like subtracting sevens backward from 100 while walking—but tend to score normally in seated balance tests.[4]

Some of my patients are more impacted by this symptom than others. If you have poor balance and frequent falls, make sure to choose exercises that are low to the ground, like the recumbent bike, and hold the handrails on the treadmill or elliptical machine when using them. Activities like yoga that involve practicing balance may be helpful, but be sure you do standing postures by a wall or other support.

One of my patients found that regular use of the Wii™ Fit Balance Board improved her balance, and that it was fun to use. These cost around $100, and have balance games and yoga postures. A few studies have found that regular use of the Balance Board improved balance and strength in other conditions.[5, 6]

We don't know exactly what causes the balance problems that often accompany fibromyalgia, but it is thought to involve poor signaling from the muscles and joints to the brain. The brain gets confused about where the body is in space. It is also possible that a brain that is distracted by all the pain signals it is getting has less capacity to devote to activities like maintaining balance.

Exercise and muscle training have been shown to improve balance in fibromyalgia, and an interesting new study found that whole-body vibration exercise helped balance. This therapy involves standing on a platform that vibrates, which stimulates muscle contraction and sensory receptors in the muscles. Subjects that received three brief episodes of low frequency vibration each week for 12 weeks had an average of 36 percent improvement in balance.[7] Other research found it helpful in improving muscle mass and balance in nursing home residents.[8]

Low blood pressure and exercise

Many people with fibromyalgia have low blood pressure that can drop even further after standing up, which must be taken into consideration while exercising. Some people can have severe drops in blood pressure leading to palpitations, dizziness and fainting. These issues are related to the effects of the chronic fight-or-flight response on blood vessels.[9]

It is important to get up slowly from any seated or laying position, especially while exercising. Eating small amounts of protein every two hours can be helpful. The most effective way I have found to treat this symptom is to drink salt water to increase your blood pressure. I tried this on the advice of my naturopath, since I was drinking 20 glasses of water a day and always feeling dehydrated and on the verge of fainting. It really helps.

Think of it is as a sports drink without the sugar. I find it actually quenches my thirst and I have to urinate less frequently throughout the day, because salt is actually what helps keep water in your bloodstream. This is why people with high blood pressure are recommended to reduce their salt consumption.

People with fibromyalgia who tend to have very low blood pressures can get some benefit from adding a little salt to their drinking water because it brings blood pressure up into the normal range. Certainly if you have high blood pressure in addition to fibromyalgia, adding salt to your water might not be safe, so use caution and discuss it with your doctor first.

There is also a prescription medication called Florinef (fludricortisone) that is sometimes used to treat severe cases of low blood pressure. This medication is a steroid that makes the kidneys retain more salt in the blood but can have many side effects, so drinking slightly salty water is probably safer.

Warm up summary

I can never remember the whole program in order, so I usually bring a list in my pocket to the gym to remind myself. Here is a list that summarizes the warm up. You can photocopy it and take it to the gym, or post it by your exercise machine at home. I highly recommend Ben Benjamin's books if you want to learn more about how to stretch, warm up, and take care of your muscles. In particular, *Exercise Without Injury* includes detailed warm-up routines to prepare for specific types of exercise.

THE WARM UP

Lie Down	Knee to Chest
Deep breaths	Thigh- Squeeze
Toe Curl	Chest-Extend-Chest-Replace
Ankle flex and circle	Chest-Extend-Lift-Replace
Foot-shake	Air-bicycle
Basic position	Shoulder Roll

CHAPTER RESOURCES

Exercise without Injury (Formerly titled *Sports without Pain*) by Ben E. Benjamin

Listen to Your Pain: The Active Person's Guide to Understanding, Identifying, and Treating Pain and Injury, by Ben E. Benjamin.

Are You Tense? The Benjamin System of Muscular Therapy: Tension Relief Through Deep Massage and Body Care, by Ben E. Benjamin

These books are available at www.benbenjamin.com and www.amazon.com.

10

IMPROVING SLEEP—
HOW TO STOP SLEEPING
WITH ONE EYE OPEN

I consider fibromyalgia to be a sleep disorder in many respects, which is why it fits so poorly into the field of rheumatology (the study of arthritis and autoimmune disease). It would fit much better into the specialty of sleep medicine. More than 95 percent of people with fibromyalgia describe their sleep as being of "poor quality."[1]

Sleep is light and unrefreshing in fibromyalgia, and followed by stiffness, aching, and fatigue in the morning. In fact, if I see a patient in my clinic who tells me they feel well rested after sleeping, I consider an alternate diagnosis.

Fibromyalgia patients often describe waking up feeling as if they were hit by a truck overnight, or "I could sleep for 24 hours straight and still wake up feeling tired." I remember waking up achy and exhausted every morning, feeling like I had run a marathon during the night.

Healthy sleep
A normal night's sleep consists of a regular pattern of dreaming and non-dreaming sleep cycles—about 4–6 complete cycles each night. The first two sleep cycles are predominated by non-dreaming deep sleep, and later cycles are mostly dreaming sleep.

Dreaming sleep is also called rapid eye movement (REM) sleep. It is the time when the brain processes memories. Many people confuse deep sleep with REM sleep, but they are two very different phases.

Deep sleep, also called stage three or slow wave, is a non-dreaming sleep in which the brain is quiet but the body is very active. It is the part of sleep that results in you feeling rested the next day. Brain waves are very slow during deep sleep, but the tissues of the body are busily undergoing healing and repair activity. Studies of marathon runners have shown that they spend more time in deep sleep after running to allow muscle tissue more recovery time. Deep sleep is also when most of the daily growth hormone secretion occurs—and as you learned in other chapters, this hormone is vital for proper muscle and tissue repair.

Children spend a lot of time in deep sleep, and thus secrete a lot of growth hormone, which makes sense because they have a lot of tissue growth to do. A child who is in deep sleep can be taken a out of their car seat, carried upstairs, and put to bed without waking up. In this deep sleep, their bodies are limp like rag dolls, but their brains are releasing huge amounts of growth hormone.

Non-dreaming sleep also has two lighter stages of sleep. Stage one the lightest stage, the transition from awake to asleep. Stage two, a slightly deeper phase of sleep, accounts for half of normal sleep time. Adults require much less deep sleep than children, but still need about 20 percent of total sleep time spent in deep sleep to be healthy.

Skimming the surface of sleep

The relationship between poor sleep and fibromyalgia has been well recognized for more than 30 years. Sleep studies consistently reveal that patients with fibromyalgia experience lighter sleep, more frequent awakenings, and not enough slow wave or deep sleep. These sleep problems do not involve the quantity of sleep, but rather the poor quality of sleep associated with abnormal sleep cycles. Fibromyalgia sleep is light, choppy, and lacking the normal prolonged periods of deep sleep.[2, 3]

Compare the two sleep pattern diagrams (pages 84–85), one showing normal sleep patterns and one from one of my patients with fibromyalgia. You can see there is a distinct difference in the deep sleep patterns. These were recorded during actual sleep studies (which are described later in the chapter).

In the fibromyalgia sleep cycle diagram, you see only a few brief choppy periods of deep sleep, frequently interrupted by a return to a lighter stage of sleep, also called a "mini-arousal." I have seen other studies of my fibromyalgia patients that actually show zero time spent in deep sleep, spending all their time in stage two or REM sleep, but never dipping down into deep sleep.

Unusual brain waves are also seen during deep sleep in people with fibromyalgia. Normally alpha brain waves should only be seen while awake, never while sleeping. But in fibromyalgia, alpha waves pop up and interrupt deep sleep, an abnormality termed alpha-delta sleep. These alpha waves are thought to reflect activation of the fight-or-flight nervous system.

Fibromyalgia Sleep

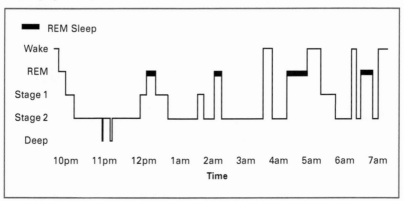

Sleep stage diagram of a person with fibromyalgia

Fibromyalgia Sleep Stage Summary

Sleep Stage	Duration (min.)	Total Sleep Time %
REM	86	23
Stage 1	49	13
Stage 2	234	63
Deep	4	1

This system, which in a healthy person is quiet during the night, has been found to be continually active during sleep in fibromyalgia. One study found the brain in fibromyalgia had twice the number or arousal/awakening episodes as healthy controls.[4] The brain in fibromyalgia undergoes hundreds of mini-arousals every night—it won't allow the body to get into deep sleep because it's trying to remain awake in order to fight off a threat.

Any factor that increases fight-or-flight nervous system activity at night is going to interfere with sleep, as anyone who has ever had caffeine or watched a horror movie just before bed can attest. Loudspeakers blaring *Danger!* all night long are not going to allow deep sleep, because your brain wants you to stay alert so you can run away or fight for your life at

Normal Sleep

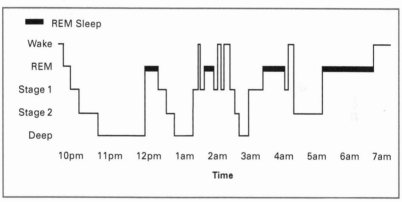

Sleep stage diagram of a normal nights sleep

Normal Sleep Stage Summary

Sleep Stage	Duration (min.)	Total Sleep Time %
REM	93	25
Stage 1	18	5
Stage 2	186	50
Deep	75	20

any moment. It was perfectly described to me by one patient as "sleeping with one eye open." Going back to our cave-woman example, in fibromyalgia the brain is staying awake to watch out for the saber-toothed tiger, even while your body is sleeping.

Inducing fibromyalgia symptoms with deep sleep deprivation

The lack of deep sleep in fibromyalgia initiates a cascade of symptoms, including fatigue and muscle pain. Studies reveal a direct relationship between poor quality sleep and other fibromyalgia symptoms such as fatigue, muscle pain, and memory and cognitive difficulties.[5] Patients notice this connection too, and tell me often that if they have a better night's sleep, they notice less muscle pain the next day.

Sleep researchers have been able to induce widespread muscle pain and fatigue in healthy volunteers simply by altering their sleep patterns to imitate those seen in fibromyalgia patients. They do this by monitoring brain waves, and just as the brain waves slow down into deep sleep, a loud noise is emitted that moves them back into a lighter stage of sleep. One study found that after three nights of deep sleep deprivation, all of the healthy young volunteers had developed sore muscles and fatigue. Essentially, they were able to induce the symptoms of fibromyalgia. Once the subjects were again allowed normal deep sleep, the muscle pain and fatigue disappeared.[6]

A more recent study on healthy middle-aged women found that deep sleep deprivation over three nights caused these healthy women to develop fatigue, muscle pain, and increased tenderness to touch. They also had an increased inflammatory flare response in the skin, suggesting a rise in inflammatory chemicals in the tissues from deep sleep deprivation. The authors of this study concluded, "These results suggest that disrupted sleep is probably an important factor in the pathophysiology of symptoms in fibromyalgia."[7]

How to improve your sleep

Increasing deep sleep and improving sleep quality can significantly improve fibromyalgia symptoms. According to Dr. Steven Berney, chief of rheumatology at Temple University: "In fibromyalgia all treatments are geared toward helping people sleep better. If we can improve their sleep, patients will get better."[8] In my practice, I see the most benefit with patients by first focusing on improving their deep sleep.

One of my initial recommendations for fibromyalgia patients is to get a sleep study to make sure there is nothing else interfering with your sleep.

SLEEP HYGIENE

BEHAVIORS AND HABITS TO IMPROVE SLEEP

Reduce caffeine. Do not have any food, drugs, or drinks that contain caffeine or other stimulants after noon.

Do not smoke within six hours before bedtime.

Do not drink alcohol within six hours before bedtime.

Do not have a heavy meal just before bedtime.

Do not do any strenuous exercise within four hours of bedtime (but exercise earlier in the day is helpful).

Body rhythms. Keep the same patterns of sleep. Go to bed at the same time and get up at the same time every day. Don't sleep in on the weekend, keep the same schedule seven days a week

Do not sleep or nap during the day, no matter how tired you are.

The bedroom should be a quiet, relaxing place to sleep.

Earplugs or a white noise machine may be useful if your room isn't quiet or you are sleeping with a snoring partner. I find the white noise produced by my bedroom HEPA machine (discussed in allergy chapter) very helpful.

Make sure the bedroom is dark with good curtains.

Don't use the bedroom for non-sleep activities such as work or eating.

Consider changing your bed if it is uncomfortable.

About half of people with fibromyalgia have an additional sleep disorder such as sleep apnea or restless legs syndrome.

A sleep study usually involves staying overnight in a sleep lab or hospital, during which your sleep is closely monitored. Machines monitor your breathing and movement during sleep, and analysis of your brain waves with EEG electrodes reveals how much time you spend in each stage of sleep. Sleep studies can be extremely informative when they reveal the poor quality of fibromyalgia sleep. I find this often helps people with fibromyalgia to understand why they are so fatigued.

Sometimes a sleep study of a fibromyalgia patient will be read as normal, only because it has no evidence for sleep apnea. In order to get the full picture in fibromyalgia, the sleep physician has to be specifically looking for the abnormal alpha waves and interrupted deep sleep of fibromyalgia. When I order a sleep study, I will often request that those aspects be focused on in detail, as they are rather subtle findings. A good quality sleep study will give you graphic information showing how much time you spent in each stage of sleep, and note the presence of any alpha-wave intrusions.

Other sleep conditions that can be observed on a sleep study include obstructive sleep apnea and restless legs syndrome. It is vital to get these evaluated and treated to eliminate any additional sleep-disrupting conditions. After diagnosing and treating any other disorders, I try to improve sleep quality with medications and behavioral changes.

Common sleep disorders that can worsen fibromyalgia sleep

Obstructive sleep apnea (OSA) is a common sleep disorder caused by soft tissue in the back of the throat collapsing and blocking the airway, resulting in the stoppage of breathing (apnea). This can occur up to 100 times an hour, and for up to one minute or more at a time. With each apnea, the brain receives a powerful arousal signal in order to trigger a breath. This can result in extremely fragmented and poor quality sleep, and profound fatigue during the day.

Usually people with sleep apnea are not aware of the multiple awakenings/arousals they experience each night, although bed partners might note loud snoring or episodes of loud gasps for air. Risk factors for OSA include obesity, smoking, thick neck, recessed chin, and a family history. However, I have definitely seen obstructive sleep apnea in people with none of these risk factors.

Treatment for obstructive sleep apnea usually involves wearing a mask that pushes oxygen into your lungs to keep your airway open, called continuous positive airway pressure (CPAP).

There is another type of sleep apnea, called central sleep apnea, that occurs when the brain "forgets" to breathe. This is most commonly seen with people taking opiates or benzodiazepine medications that affect the breathing regulation centers of the brain. Central sleep apnea is treated by changing medications.

Restless legs syndrome (RLS) is a neurological disorder characterized by uncomfortable sensations in the legs, often described as burning, creeping, tugging, or insects crawling. Lying down and trying to relax activates the symptoms, and kicking or moving the legs give temporary relief. As a result, most people with RLS have difficulty falling asleep and staying asleep.

RLS occurs in both genders, although the incidence is slightly higher in women. Most patients who are severely affected are middle-aged or older. In addition, the severity of the disorder appears to increase with age. RLS usually responds very well to medications that increase dopamine levels, such as ropirinole and pramipexole.

Sleep medications

Unfortunately, most sedative medications do not change the abnormal sleep patterns seen in fibromyalgia. None of the commonly prescribed sleep medications like zolpidem (Ambien), eszopiclone (Lunesta), or clonazepam (Klonopin) improve sleep quality. Studies of these sleep medications have not found any improvement in fibromyalgia symptoms.[9-11] Most sedative medications simply induce sleep and do not affect brainwave patterns while sleeping. You just get more of whatever sleep you would usually get, which in fibromyalgia is pretty poor quality.

None of these sleeping medications are strong enough to overwhelm the blaring loudspeakers of the brain in fibromyalgia and stop the alphawave intrusions into deep sleep. While they don't address the fundamental sleep problem, they do treat insomnia and can keep you asleep a little longer, which can sometimes be helpful.

Complicating matters further, commonly prescribed opiate-based pain medications such as morphine or oxycodone have actually been shown to have a negative impact on deep sleep. One study showed that morphine given to healthy individuals decreased the amount of deep sleep significantly from the usual 20 percent of total sleep to only 6 percent.[12] This sleep disturbance may explain why opiate-based pain medications like morphine have not been found to be helpful overall in fibromyalgia.

Interestingly, two of the medications that have shown some benefit for pain in fibromyalgia do have a mild effect on sleep quality. In some studies, both pregabalin (Lyrica) and gabapentin (Neurontin) show slightly increased time spent in deep sleep, and that may explain some of their effectiveness in fibromyalgia.[13]

However, there is a new medicine awaiting FDA approval for use in fibromyalgia that has been shown to improve deep sleep. This medication is a strong sedative medicine related to gamma-hydroxybutyrate (GHB) that was originally developed in the 1960s to put people to sleep for surgery. Researchers noticed that it seemed to induce a period of deep sleep, from which people awoke feeling refreshed. This later was developed into a related drug called sodium oxybate (Xyrem') that increases both the time spent in deep sleep and secretion of growth hormone. Giving this drug to rats increases levels of growth hormone and also speeds up wound healing.[14]

In 2002, the FDA approved sodium oxybate for use in narcolepsy, a neurological disorder in which the brain cannot regulate sleep/wake cycles. Thus, people with narcolepsy fall asleep unpredictably throughout the day, and wake up frequently all night long. A sleep pattern diagram of someone with narcolepsy actually looks similar to that of fibromyalgia, with choppy interrupted deep sleep. In narcolepsy, this medication has been shown to condense fragmented sleep cycles, increase time in deep, slow-wave sleep and reduce nighttime awakenings.

Sodium oxybate is an unusual medication because it is a liquid, has a rapid onset of action, and only lasts in the body for two to four hours. It has to be given in two different doses, with the first at bedtime and the second a few hours later. This allows for two good quality deep sleep cycles, which essentially replicates what occurs in normal sleep.

This medication works by binding with certain receptors in the brain called GABA receptors, which induces a general reduction in brain activity. In particular, it slows activity in the areas of the brain controlling the fight-or-flight response and temporarily shuts off this response and allows for deep sleep. Normally the fight-or-flight system should be off-line while we sleep, but as you know in fibromyalgia that is not the case. Sodium oxybate forces the fight-or-flight system to shut down, allowing for deep sleep.

Several studies have examined sodium oxybate in fibromyalgia, and all have shown improvement in sleep patterns, fatigue, and pain. Two groups compared sleep studies before and during treatment and found that sodium oxybate significantly increased deep sleep and reduced alpha-wave intrusion. At the start of one study, the average fibromyalgia subject experienced 14.9 percent deep sleep (as a percentage of total sleep time) compared to a normal 20 percent. After using the medication nightly for one month, the sleep study was repeated and this time the percentage of deep sleep had increased to 21.5 percent. There were also notably fewer alpha waves seen during deep sleep. Pain and fatigue were also significantly reduced in the group taking the medication. In contrast the placebo group had no change in the amount of deep sleep or alpha waves.[15, 16]

A much larger randomized study done at multiple medical centers found that eight weeks of sodium oxybate use improved fibromyalgia symptoms. There was a notable reduction in symptoms of both pain and fatigue compared to those taking placebo; almost one third of the sodium oxybate patients reported a 50 percent reduction in pain.[17] A European study found that two-thirds of the fibromyalgia subjects taking this medication experienced a significant reduction in pain and fatigue.[18]

This is very exciting, because these are much better results than from any currently available medication for fibromyalgia. In narcolepsy, it takes about three months of regular use to reach maximal benefit. Since the fibromyalgia studies only looked at eight weeks of use, there is potential that with longer use it could be even more effective.

It would be very interesting know whether using sodium oxybate to improve sleep quality could reduce the cognitive difficulties known as "fibrofog," but this has not yet been studied. One of the leading researchers in the field of cognition in fibromyalgia has found that fibromyalgia subjects perform the same as healthy people who have been deprived of sleep. In particular, just like people who are artificially deprived of sleep in an experiment, people with fibromyalgia have a harder time with word recall and multi-tasking. So the poor memory and difficulty multi-tasking that is seen in fibromyalgia may simply be a reflection of deep sleep deprivation.

In my personal experience taking sodium oxybate, I found it dramatically reduced my fatigue, and I woke up feeling rested and ready to go, without that familiar dragging, achy feeling. Mentally, I felt sharper, and I had more energy during the day and less "brain fog." Most importantly, it also reduced my pain, and in particular I noticed that repetitive motion did not cause as much pain and my body seemed to bounce back quicker from injury or exercise. I also was able to tolerate more prolonged and intense exercise.

I definitely found that taking the two doses of medication each night (one at bedtime and one a few hours later) was necessary to feel the full benefit. But even though it was not one long uninterrupted sleep, it was very refreshing. It is the quality of the sleep that matters more than the quantity.

My family also noticed a change in me while I was taking this medication. As most people with fibromyalgia do, I frequently modified my activities to limit pain without even thinking about it. For example, I always spread out the groceries into many smaller loads, rather than carrying a heavy grocery bag into the house.

After about six weeks of using sodium oxybate, I went on a trip with my mother, who has limited mobility due to arthritis. Without thinking, as we were disembarking from the airplane, I grabbed both her heavy carry-on suitcase and mine, and carried them both off the airplane. My mom pointed out what I had just done, and I realized that my arms had not hurt when I lifted those heavy bags and carried them more than 100 feet, and I didn't get the usual increased pain after exertion that I am so used to. My husband noticed that I had much more energy to play with our daughter, and that I was doing more things like lifting her up and swinging her around that normally I just wouldn't do because of the painful consequences later. And those consequences didn't come! It was amazing.

Even more impressive was the fibromyalgia patient that walked in to my office after three months of sodium oxybate treatment who told me her pain was gone. This was absolutely one of the best moments of my medical career. Another patient recently told me that she feels "not perfect, but so much better" since starting the medication.

Unfortunately, I have not been able to prescribe it for very many of my patients, because, as of the writing of this book, this medication has not been approved for use in fibromyalgia by the FDA. It is extremely expensive (around $20,000 per year), and is generally not covered by insurance for fibromyalgia since it is not FDA-approved for this condition. Thus my experience has been limited to a handful of patients.

Of the few I have prescribed it for, some had impressive results, but others did not tolerate it due to side effects. The most common side effects are nausea, headache, and dizziness. It very rarely can cause bedwetting, because in a deep sleep signals from the bladder might not wake you up.

It certainly is unlike any other medication experience. After I take a dose at night, I feel a little light-headed and spacey, but not really sleepy, for about 30 minutes. I read or watch TV during this time, and it is not unpleasant, just a bit odd. It's a little like how I feel after I have blown up too many balloons. Then suddenly I feel intensely sleepy, and within seconds I am asleep, often without even enough time to turn off the light or taking off my glasses. Then three or four hours later I wake up and take the second dose, and when I wake up in the morning I feel ready to go.

There are some additional challenges when it comes to prescribing sodium oxybate due to its relation to GHB, a controlled substance that gained notoriety in the bar and club scene as a "date-rape drug" when slipped into an alcoholic beverage. Of course, these instances involved very high doses combined with other sedatives like alcohol. Just like opiate-based pain medications, sodium oxybate does have the potential for addiction or abuse. When combined with other sedatives, such as alcohol, opiate pain medications, or benzodiazepines, it can result in potentially deadly levels of respiratory suppression or even death. That said, studies have shown sodium oxybate is safe when used in low-doses under medical supervision.

In attempt to prevent abuse and misuse of sodium oxybate, it is distributed directly by a central pharmacy associated with the drug company. It is then sent to your house via overnight mail. It is recommended that this medication be avoided in patients with history of drug abuse or alcoholism. And it should not be prescribed to anyone who is currently taking any sedating medication such as opiate-based pain medications or benzodiazepines. This can be challenging because many fibromyalgia patients do take opiate pain medications, and these would need to be stopped before using sodium oxybate. Also it cannot be combined with alcohol, as this can cause excess sedation and reduced breathing. It also has a risk of worsening sleep apnea, but is felt to be safe to use when obstructive sleep apnea is being adequately treated with a CPAP mask. For this reason, some doctors order a sleep study prior to prescribing sodium oxybate to evaluate for sleep apnea.

While sodium oxybate can help normalize deep sleep and growth hormone, it can't fix all the problems in fibromyalgia as long as the fight-or-flight nervous system is still in overdrive. The problems with fascial tension, leaky gut, and inflammation remain. However, I think use of this medication, in combination with myofascial release, exercise, and dietary changes can result in impressive improvement of fibromyalgia symptoms.

CHAPTER RESOURCES

For more information on sodium oxybate, see www.xyrem.com.

A very good resource to learn more about sleep is http://healthysleep.med.harvard.edu/healthy/science.

11

MANUAL THERAPY FOR YOUR FASCIA

I never had much improvement in pain after getting a conventional massage, sometimes feeling even more achy and tired afterward. I tried many styles of massage, but it was only after stumbling upon myofascial release (MFR) therapy that I found significant pain relief. My patients that have tried this therapy also find it helpful; one said, "Myofascial release works better than any pill to relieve my pain."

MFR is quite different from traditional massage therapy, which consists of repeated stroking of muscles in order to promote overall relaxation. Instead, MFR focuses on manipulating and stretching the fascia, the dense connective tissue that surrounds, infiltrates, and supports the musculoskeletal system.

If you were to gently bend your head to the side right now, as if trying to rest your ear on your shoulder, you will feel a pulling or stretching sensation on the opposite side of your neck, from your shoulder up to your jaw. What you are feeling is not actually stretching of the muscle—there is no one muscle that runs from your shoulder to your ear—but stretching of the fascia surrounding all the muscles between your jaw and your shoulder. The fascia covers and connects every muscle in your body. If a myofascial release practitioner were to put one hand on your shoulder and one near your jaw, this gentle stretching of the fascia can actually break up adhesions and "sticky" areas.

Myofascial release and Rolfing™

The primary manual therapies that address the fascia are myofascial release (MFR) and Rolfing˚. A form of hands-on manipulation and movement education developed more than 50 years ago, Rolfing works especially on the fascia around the joints. This technique focuses on correcting posture and joint alignment in a series of 10–12 sessions, with a goal of correcting unhealthy movement and tissue patterns.

MFR is a related technique that focuses more on the fascia surrounding the muscles. It utilizes a combination of sustained manual traction and prolonged gentle stretching maneuvers to break up adhesions in the fascia. Essentially the therapist slowly and gently stretches the fascia to break up "sticky" areas of excess collagen cross-links that are called adhesions or restrictions.

The specific technique depends on which part of the body is being treated. Over flat surfaces of the body (chest, back, abdomen) the cross hand release is performed. In this technique the therapist steadies the fascia with one hand and then crosses the opposite hand over the fixed hand. Gentle downward pressure is applied and the hands are moved apart until a point of resistance is encountered. This is a point of fascial contracture and force is maintained at this point for 2–3 minutes until release is accomplished. This is distinctly different from the stroking-type techniques used in standard massage.

Unfortunately, the term "myofascial release" has become widely and inappropriately used as a generic term for massage, and many practitioners claiming to use these techniques are actually just performing deep-tissue massage. But myofascial release involves prolonged stretching of the fascia and is very different from deep-tissue massage. When I refer to MFR in this chapter, I am referring specifically to the specialized technique originated by a physical therapist named John Barnes. See the chapter resources for information on how to find a therapist trained in this technique.

How does myofascial release work?

The fascia is actually a very dense gel that with slow and sustained pressure can be molded and stretched.[1] MFR breaks up the microadhesions and scarring in the fascia, which in my opinion are the source of pain in fibromyalgia (as discussed in Chapter 5). By addressing these painful areas of the fascia, myofascial release therapy can reduce pain.[2] One scientist writes, "We know that there are many sensory receptors, including pain receptors in fascia, which points our attention in fibromyalgia and other kinds of soft-tissue pain syndromes to a much higher value of therapeutic interventions in the fascia itself."[3]

The fascia has many different layers. For ideal muscle health and movement, these layers need to glide over one another very smoothly. But excess scar tissue or collagen connections between the layers can make them "sticky" and restrict movement. Fibrosis and adhesions in the fascia in one area of the body can affect other parts, much like pulling on a piece of yarn in a sweater can cause tightness in the sweater very distant from where you are pulling. When you pull the string, it not only causes a localized knot, it can affect the shape of the whole sweater, just as fascial restrictions can effect other parts of the body and even whole body posture.

The effects of MFR can result in long-term changes in the tissue. A fascinating study on patients with carpal tunnel syndrome found that myofascial release not only reduced pain, but actually produced documented increased diameter of the carpal tunnel on magnetic resonance imaging.[4] Another study reported that MFR therapy reduced post-radiation chest wall tenderness from fibrosis and adhesions in breast cancer patients.[5]

No studies on MFR in fibromyalgia have yet been published, but I am hoping to change that. I am leading a pilot study at Oregon Health and Sciences University to compare this technique to standard massage therapy in fibromyalgia.

Some studies that have used techniques similar to MFR have shown reduced pain in fibromyalgia. One study found that osteopathic manipulative techniques that incorporated MFR techniques reduced fibromyalgia symptoms more than medications alone.[6] Connective tissue massage— a European manual therapy that is related to myofascial release—also showed a pain-relieving benefit in fibromyalgia.[7]

Treating the fascia in fibromyalgia

In 1904, Dr. Ralph Stockman, a Scottish physician, wrote that the pain of chronic rheumatism (what we now call fibromyalgia) was due to thickenings that developed in the fibrous connective tissue of muscle. He recognized the importance of manual therapy in treating this condition and noted that thickened fibrous tissue could only be removed by "local and well-directed manipulations."[8]

Current research lends support to Dr. Stockman's theory of abnormalities in the fascia in patients with fibromyalgia, and to the effectiveness of manual therapies. There is growing evidence that therapies such as MFR can break up excess collagen adhesions and reduce pain and tension in the tissue.[9, 10] In addition, fibroblasts that undergo sustained tissue pressure, like that administered during MFR, become activated and secrete chemicals that accelerate the healing process.[11]

MFR may also have a direct calming influence on the fight-or-flight system activation seen in fibromyalgia. As you know, the fascia contains many nerve endings, with some sensing pain and some sensing pressure. It also contains nerve endings from the fight-or-flight nervous system. One specific type of nerve ending in the fascia responds to gentle sustained pressure by lowering the activity of the fight-or-flight nervous system.[12]

A study found a reduction in the fight-or-flight nervous system effects after myofascial release was applied to pelvic muscles. Interestingly, this resulted in reduced fight-or-flight activity both during the session and for 24 hours afterwards as well.[13] As discussed previously, the fascia and fight-or-flight nervous system seem to have a direct connection. According to one expert, "Any intervention on the fascia is also an intervention on the autonomic nervous system."[14]

What does MFR feel like?

It is nothing like a massage, although afterwards I always felt incredibly relaxed. It is slow, gentle, and sustained pressure on your tissue. Sometimes it feels like a gentle stretching or pulling, and other times it can be a more painful friction sensation, almost like a rug burn. But overall, the experience is pleasant, and afterwards I feel so much less pain that I am almost willing to endure anything. After very intense sessions, I have felt a little sore the next day, but it was usually minimal.

Most of the subjects in my study on MFR were able to correctly identify which treatment they were receiving, even though they were not told. One subject in the MFR group said, "I don't know what that was, but it was definitely not a massage."

In the beginning, I had pretty intensive MFR work over a period of a few months, and found improvement in my pain levels, particularly in my back, neck, and jaw areas. I also noted definite changes in the way my body felt. I started to feel my tissues relaxing. I slept better. Looking back on it now, the MFR helped my body reduce some fight-or-flight nervous system influence and helped my tissues to actually unlock or relax. For a few days after a session, I definitely noticed a difference in my baseline level of muscle tension.

After those intensive few months where I got as much MFR as I could (sometimes 6–8 hours a week), I then started getting it weekly, then monthly, and now I just require occasional "tune-ups."

Most MFR practitioners will take pictures of your posture in the beginning, to both help direct treatment and document progress. I was astonished at my posture and the changes about eight sessions of MFR produced. In the before pictures, my pelvis is tilted forward and my head protrudes forward over my chest. After six months, my posture was visibly improved, with my head, neck, and pelvis aligned normally.

What is myofascial pain syndrome?

Myofascial pain syndrome is a name for a focal area of restrictions and pain in the fascia, usually limited to one or two muscle groups. The fascia becomes inflamed and restrictions and pain develop. This is similar to what is seen in fibromyalgia, but just in a much more localized area of the fascia.

In fibromyalgia, restrictions and pain are caused by the stress response tightening of the fascia and lack of growth hormone and deep sleep. In focal myofascial pain syndromes, the restrictions occur as a result of injury or repetitive motion, poor posture, or poor body mechanics. Certainly those same factors can also contribute to fascial injury in someone with fibromyalgia. The widespread tissue tension makes people with fibromyalgia more much more prone to developing particular "hot spots" in the fascia, particularly in the jaw and pelvis.

As you learned in earlier chapters, when the fight-or-flight response is activated, the muscles and fascia of the body tighten in a protective response. In particular, the jaw and pelvis are where we tend to tense to brace for an attack. That tightening of the fascia is a normal response to danger, but when it happens constantly it can lead to adhesions and pain.

When myofascial pain occurs in the jaw area it is called temporomandibular joint dysfunction (TMD or TMJ). This is a collective term for clinical problems involving the jaw muscles and joint. TMD is the most common pain condition treated by dentists and affects about one third of the general population. Symptoms can include jaw, ear, and neck pain, restricted mouth opening, and joint clicking or popping with movement.

Some cases of TMD are primarily related to dental issues, misalignment of the jaw, or arthritis of the joint. However, most cases are due to fascial restrictions in the jaw muscles that can be from clenching the jaw or grinding the teeth, and not primarily from issues in the joint itself. In fact, dentists often separate this disorder into two groups: TMD that originates from the joint, and TMD that comes from the muscles and fascia.

TMD is very common in fibromyalgia; between 75–94 percent of people with fibromyalgia also have jaw pain or "masticatory myofascial pain syndrome."[15, 16] It is not surprising that if you have widespread fascial pain and restrictions, as in fibromyalgia, this would also affect the fascia around the jaw.

Myofascial release can be very helpful in reducing TMD pain. The treatment usually involves releases inside the mouth, around the ears, and in the low back and pelvis. There is a definite relationship between the jaw and the pelvis, maybe because we tend to clench them both. I was surprised by how much my jaw was helped when MFR was done on my pelvic floor muscles. Unfortunately, no studies so far have looked directly at this therapy in jaw pain but, anecdotally, many of my patients have also found it helpful.

Chronic pelvic pain is another very common focal myofascial pain syndrome. Symptoms can include bladder pain and pelvic pain, frequent urination, and painful intercourse. Research supports the concept that increased tone and tension in the pelvic floor muscles are present in this condition, and it often responds dramatically to therapies directed at the fascia. One pelvic pain study found that 57 percent of subjects treated with MFR had moderate to marked improvement, compared to only 21 percent in the group receiving standard massage.[17] Another study described significant reduction in pain during intercourse after treatment with pelvic myofascial release techniques, and more than half of the subjects were able to return to pain-free intercourse.[18]

What about myofascial trigger points?

Myofascial trigger points are defined as "a hyperirritable spot, usually within a taut band of skeletal muscle or in the muscle fascia which is painful on compression and can give rise to characteristic referred pain."[19] They are very common, and can occur in any muscle that is under strain in the human body. In fact, almost everyone has a trigger point in the trapezius and upper back muscles when under stress.

Theories vary as to what actually causes trigger points. The most popular theory is that dysfunction of the junction where nerves meet the muscle causes an abnormal contraction in one small area of the muscle. Increased electrical activity in trigger points compared to surrounding muscle has been demonstrated and supports this theory.[20]

So far the contribution of the fascia to the development of myofascial trigger points has been pretty much neglected in research. Even though the word fascia is right there in the name, all the research focus has been on the "myo" or muscle cells contribution.

In my opinion, myofascial trigger points are "hot spots" of fascia that irritate nearby muscle cells causing them to abnormally contract in certain areas. Trigger points are often noted to develop after injury, mechanical stress, or repetitive micro-trauma—all conditions under which fascia becomes "sticky." This combination of contracted muscle cells and sticky fascia creates the taut, painful lump or band that is a myofascial trigger point.

Since the fascia in fibromyalgia is already contracted and irritable, it is very easy to develop these hot spots, and trigger points are quite common. Treating myofascial trigger points can be very helpful in reducing local muscle pain. The most effective treatments for trigger points are those that involve physically disrupting the tissue by stretching, massage, or insertion of a needle into the muscle. Think about that snag in a sweater, and the bunching or knot of fibers that it causes. The only way to unravel the knot is to pull the fibers away from each other and slide them back in place. A trigger point is essentially a snag in the fiber of the fascia, and these sticky fibers need to be physically broken up to allow the muscle to relax.

Myofascial trigger points can be treated by inserting needles to break up the knot, either with injection of medicines or without. Focused, intense finger pressure on a trigger point, and some other massage techniques can also undo the contraction knot. Myofascial release can also be quite effective in breaking up trigger points, but certain very irritable or deep knots do benefit from trigger point injections in my experience.

Deep frictioning therapy
Although MFR breaks up adhesions in the connective tissue that wraps around the muscles, it is not as effective at treating adhesions and scars in the tendons. Tendons are short, dense strips of connective tissue that connect muscle to bone. The fascia around the muscle becomes denser towards the end of the muscle and forms the tendon. Since a tendon is short and dense it is difficult to stretch and a different approach is needed.

When I developed a repetitive stress injury in my arms (elbow tendinitis), it seemed to be the only thing MFR could not help me with, and the pain persisted until I found a technique called deep frictioning therapy.

Deep frictioning is a technique developed by Dr. James Cyriax, a British orthopedic physician who did pioneering work in the field of musculoskeletal injury. This technique involves strumming back and forth over the fibers of the tendon (perpendicular to the fibers of the tendon, like strumming a guitar string) that helps break up scar tissue in the tendon and allow for healing of the injury. A related therapy, the Graston technique, utilizes metal instruments to apply the friction.

When the body lays down scar tissue in response to an injury, it does so in a hurried and haphazard way. If you were to look at a healthy tendon under a microscope, you would see tissue that is neatly organized with rows of collagen fibers. However, a tendon that is repairing from an injury would show collagen fibers in all sorts of directions, almost like a pile of cooked spaghetti. Gradually, the body then remodels the scar tissue and gets it to line up in organized rows again.

However, in the case of a repetitive stress injury, the tendon never has a chance to get to the remodeling phase because it is continually getting reinjured, so it just keeps laying down more and more haphazardly arranged collagen. Unfortunately, this haphazardly arranged scar tissue is a weaker tissue and more prone to re-injury, and can generate significant pain. Thus you can see how a repetitive stress injury can become quite a chronic problem, with continual re-injury of poorly formed scar tissue.

Friction therapy can help align the collagen fibers correctly and promote tendon healing. For me, after about eight sessions of rather painful friction therapy on the tendons of my forearms, my elbow tendinitis was much improved.

I do want to say another word about a therapy I tried for inflamed tendons that did not help me and was quite expensive. Prolotherapy involves the injection of a dextrose solution (sugar water) into the injured tendon. This theoretically causes a localized inflammation in the tendon to increase the blood supply and flow of nutrients and stimulate tissue repair. I read a great deal about this technique before I tried it, and the principle behind it is quite intriguing. There are a few small studies that did show benefit from prolotherapy in elbow tendinitis,[21] but I did not find it helpful. It might help in other conditions, but it may not be able to stimulate an adequate tissue response in fibromyalgia.

I highly recommend that people with fibromyalgia seek out manual therapy that focuses on the fascia, whether that is Rolfing, MFR, or friction massage. Most MFR practitioners have completed extensive advanced training, and thus the treatments can be costly relative to standard massage. Sometimes insurance will pay for some of the cost of this type of therapy.

Certainly, manual therapy is a much better place to focus your resources compared to some of the expensive, but ineffective, supplements often promoted for fibromyalgia.

CHAPTER RESOURCES

To learn more about the John Barnes MFR technique and to find a therapist in your area, visit www.myofascialrelease.com.

Healing Ancient Wounds: The Renegade's Wisdom by John Barnes

To learn more about Rolfing, or find a therapist in your area visit www.rolf.org.

To learn more about friction therapy: *Listen to Your Pain: The Active Person's Guide to Understanding, Identifying, and Treating Pain and Injury* by Ben E. Benjamin.

12

REDUCING THE FIGHT-OR-FLIGHT RESPONSE

People with fibromyalgia often startle easily, practically jumping out of their skin with any loud noise. One patient described how she felt like she was a combat veteran, even though she had never seen combat.

When the autonomic nervous system is stuck in the fight-or-flight response, the brain is priming the body to instantly respond to any danger. This can translate into an intense awareness of your surroundings. A friend with fibromyalgia described herself as a "heavy receiver," and I notice my own body tensing when I watch a stranger struggling to find bus change or arguing with someone. I have to remind myself, *That is not my stress.*

The constant fight-or-flight response in the body makes it very difficult to fall asleep or have sex, both bodily functions that requires the brain to let down its guard and allow the rest-and-digest nervous system to take over. In fibromyalgia, in order to get into the rest-and-digest mode we have to overcome the incredible dominance of the fight-or-flight response. It sometimes feels like I cannot take a deep enough breath to relax my body. One person with fibromyalgia told me: "Every time I check in with my body, I am aware of muscle tightness. I consciously try to relax my body, but as soon as I am not thinking about it anymore, my body goes right back to clenching."

We have not yet found a way to reverse fight-or-flight dominance in fibromyalgia permanently. Once we find that, I think we will have discovered the cure to fibromyalgia. The best we can do now is treat the problems caused by fight-or-flight dominance and try to encourage the nervous system to shift into rest-and-digest mode as frequently as possible, even if just for short periods of time.

Due to the strong fight-or-flight dominance in fibromyalgia, it can be harder to get into the relaxation response, but it can be done. Anything you can do to induce more of a parasympathetic state, even temporarily, will help. The parasympathetic state is where your body does its very important rest-and-digest functions, and in fibromyalgia, the goal is to give your body as much time in the parasympathetic state as possible. Even if it is only temporary, it can still be beneficial.

I have found it is possible to get into the rest-and-digest mode, but it is a battle requiring continued and repeated effort on my part. It will take me almost an hour of a massage until I feel any shift into relaxation in my body, and almost as soon as the massage is over I find myself back in the tensed fight-or-flight mode. It takes me a long time to relax enough to sleep. In fibromyalgia, it takes significant effort to reduce the effects if the fight-or-flight response even temporarily. The challenge here is that the parts of the brain running the stress response are not under conscious control.

I want to emphasize here that you did not "think" your way into the fight-or-flight response, and you can't think your way out of it. The stress response is controlled by a deep, primal part of your brain that is below the level of conscious thought. This is the part of your brain that is controlling your heart rate and blood pressure and digestion while you read this—all functions that don't require or respond to conscious thought. You can't think your way into having a bowel movement, it just happens automatically.

This primal part of your brain only listens to signals from the body. In order to use conscious thought to affect the stress response, you have to change the signals that your body is sending to the brain. The best way to consciously affect the autonomic nervous system is through controlling your breathing. Breathing is the only bodily function that we do both consciously and unconsciously. By changing your breath into slow, deep breathing, you can actually directly stimulate the rest-and-digest nervous system.

This results in the relaxation response—essentially the opposite of the fight-or-flight response. Herbert Benson, a pioneering mind-body researcher, wrote a book called *The Relaxation Response* in 1975 that describes various techniques to induce this response. Anytime you affect your breathing consciously you can induce the relaxation response. Other ways include meditation, yoga, and guided muscle relaxation. Biofeedback therapy uses muscle monitors to promote awareness of where you are holding muscles tight and help you focus on relaxing muscle tension.

I personally have not had much success with meditation, and in fact whenever I try to just "observe my breath," I seem to almost hyperventilate. I do much better, and can get into the relaxation response more easily, by doing yoga, which combines deep breathing with movement and stretching. I also find that myofascial release activates the relaxation response in my body (read more about this in Chapter 11).

But each person is different, and what works for me might not work for you. I strongly encourage you to experiment and find what works to induce your relaxation response. Regardless of the method you use, it is essential to guide your body there as often as you can. In fibromyalgia, this needs to be a continual, daily effort to reduce the fight-or-flight response and its negative effects on the body as much as possible

Since we don't consciously control the fight-or-flight response, we can't think it away. But every time you become aware of the tightness of your muscles, try taking a few slow, deep breaths. I find that focusing on unclenching my pelvic muscles naturally leads me to loosen the clenching in my jaw, low back, and stomach. When you consciously take some deep breaths and unclench your muscles, it sends a signal to your brain to shift away from fight-or-flight mode.

There are two other interesting therapies that may be able to affect the brain directly and encourage a shift into the relaxation response.

Cranial electrotherapy stimulation
This is a technique that reportedly can activate the parasympathetic nervous system in the brain. It was developed in the U.S.S.R. in the 1950s as

a sleep inducer (it was called electrosleep at the time), and was heavily researched in the U.S. in the 1970s as a treatment for anxiety.

Basically, this therapy involves the use of microcurrent levels of electricity transmitted the head between an electrode placed on each ear. The level of electricity is so low it is often not detectable to the user. It has been shown in some studies to induce a state of relaxation, a sense of calm or clear-headedness.

One study found that a session of cranial electrotherapy stimulation (CES) reduced anxiety and muscle tension as effectively as a session of guided relaxation.[1] Another found that it shifted the brain-wave patterns seen on an EEG to those associated with parasympathetic, relaxed states. Other studies have shown that using CES can help people with insomnia fall asleep faster. A Russian study and a small study in the U.S. showed that CES therapy did cause changes in heart rate, skin temperature, and muscle tension consistent with increased parasympathetic activity.[2, 3]

How could low-dose electricity applied to the brain affect the parasympathetic nervous system? The truth is, no one knows for sure. One theory is that the electricity passing between the ears hits the vagus nerve, a branch of which runs near the ear. The vagus nerve is the main conduit of signals in the parasympathetic nervous system from the brain to the body. Others think the electric current runs through the areas of the brain that control the autopilot nervous system and that this shifts the brain signals more towards a parasympathetic mode. Another suggestion is that the electrical current acts as a rhythmic pacemaker throughout the brain, changing brainwave patterns to a slower, more relaxed rhythm.

Could this therapy be beneficial in fibromyalgia? Possibly. Two different, well-designed placebo-controlled studies showed reduction in pain and anxiety symptoms in fibromyalgia with CES treatment. One of the studies reported an almost 30 percent improvement in tender point scores (which measure how many tender points hurt when pressed) and in self-reported pain scores in fibromyalgia patients using real CES treatment compared to "sham" CES therapy.[4, 5]

One way CES therapy could be theoretically beneficial in fibromyalgia is if it could transition the brain to a more parasympathetic state while sleeping, resulting in more deep sleep and less alpha-wave intrusion. A study done in the 1970s noted slightly increased time spent in deep sleep in healthy people using CES therapy every day for three weeks. This has not yet been studied for improving deep sleep in fibromyalgia patients, but hopefully it will be.[6]

I tried using CES therapy for about a month myself, for 30 minutes a day. At higher settings it gave me a headache, and I could feel a prickly sensation in my ears. But at the lowest setting (the level they used in studies because it is below the level of sensation), I found it very relaxing, and it helped me to fall asleep quicker. I think it might have helped my sleep a little, but I certainly did not notice a dramatic effect. After a month of daily use, I did not notice any reduction in pain or fatigue.

But I did feel very clear-headed after a CES session, and I felt I was a little bit sharper during that month. And this led me to do some reading on one other area where this therapy might benefit people with fibromyalgia: cognition. One of the more challenging symptoms of fibromyalgia is the "fibrofog," the poor memory, reduced attention span, and difficulty multi-tasking that everyone reading this book who has fibromyalgia will probably recognize. I personally think that fibrofog is caused by the years and years of deep sleep deprivation seen in fibromyalgia. Interestingly, healthy people who are sleep-deprived score and people with fibromyalgia score very similarly on tests of memory and attention.

But other than getting more deep sleep, what can be done about impaired cognition in fibromyalgia? There is some evidence that CES can improve cognition in other conditions. In long-term alcoholics, three weeks of daily CES therapy was noted to improve short-term memory.[7] Patients with complaints of difficulty focusing on tasks (what we now label attention deficit disorder) performed better on IQ testing after three weeks of CES.[8]

Certainly, more research needs to be done on CES in fibromyalgia. Does it actually induce a parasympathetic state as measured by heart-rate variability? Could it result in increased deep sleep and better cognition? Unfortunately, it is rather expensive. A CES device can cost between $400–500. But if further research shows a real measurable benefit of CES therapy in fibromyalgia, then it might be worth a try, in my opinion.

Craniosacral therapy

Craniosacral therapy is a manual therapy technique developed from the osteopathic medical tradition almost 100 years ago, and further developed by Dr. John Upledger in the 1980s. The basic premise of this therapy is that the fluid around the brain and spinal cord, called the cerebrospinal fluid, has rhythmic pulsations. These pulsations can be interpreted—and altered—by a therapist who places their hands at the base of the skull and spine and does gentle manipulations.

I have experienced craniosacral therapy as part of a massage or myofascial release session, and it is incredibly calming and relaxing. Usually, the base of my skull is resting on the therapist's hands, and with very slight movements of their hands I start to feel very sleepy and heavy, similar to the feeling when you first slip into a hot bath. I have actually almost fallen asleep multiple times while having craniosacral therapy performed, and the relaxation lingers after the session, too.

Is there any science behind this? Images obtained from magnetic resonance imaging have helped to ascertain that both the cerebrospinal fluid and brain move in a pulsatile manner within the cranium, and these pulses are affected by the movement of breathing and of blood in the vessels.[9-11] In addition, the nerves of the parasympathetic nervous system exit the spinal cord at the top near the base of the skull (cranium) and at the bottom near the tailbone (sacrum), which is why it is sometimes called the craniosacral nervous system.

Could gentle pressure on the top and bottom of the spine somehow affect the parasympathetic nervous system to promote a more relaxed state of being? That certainly seems reasonable to me, although as far as I can tell no studies have been done to prove this. I wonder if this is how deep breathing might act to enhance the parasympathetic nervous system, by affecting the pulses in the CSF, similar to a therapist's gentle touch.

Emotional and spiritual healing: Feeling safe in the world again

Survivors of trauma suffer from higher rates of depression, anxiety, and eating and substance abuse disorders than the general population.[12] Unfortunately, as you have learned in prior chapters, many people diagnosed with fibromyalgia have suffered a major trauma in their lives. One study found that 90 percent of women with fibromyalgia reported being physically or sexually assaulted in their lifetime. And a quarter of those with fibromyalgia also have post-traumatic stress disorder, an anxiety disorder characterized by nightmares, recurrent memories of traumatic events, and avoidance behaviors.[13]

Compared to other chronic illnesses, fibromyalgia is more often accompanied by depression and anxiety. One large study found 60 percent of subjects with fibromyalgia met a diagnosis for major depression, compared to 28 percent of rheumatoid arthritis subjects.[14] Since both depression and fibromyalgia seem to run in families, some researchers theorize that there may be similar genes that increase risk for both conditions. Certainly depression and other psychiatric disorders are complex conditions related to brain biochemistry, genetics, and many other factors.

However the higher rates of psychiatric disorders in fibromyalgia may also be due in part to the association with trauma. Not everyone with fibromyalgia is clinically depressed, and depression most definitely does not cause fibromyalgia. But it is important to recognize that the experience of trauma makes one more prone to anxiety and depression, which make it even harder to deal with the overwhelming fatigue and muscle pain of fibromyalgia.

A stress response system stuck in fight-or-flight mode leads not only to the physical symptoms of fibromyalgia, but is also experienced emotionally as a feeling of unease. This can intensify the experience of depression and cause a general sense of anxiety. Even fibromyalgia patients who never experienced a trauma often describe vague feelings of anxiety and unease. A friend described it as "just never feeling safe." This is directly related, in my opinion, to the emotional experience of a brain being stuck in the fight-or-flight response.

We don't have a way—yet—to flip the stress response switch back. We do have effective treatments and medications that can help with many of the physical symptoms of fibromyalgia. We also have psychiatric medications and talk therapy to address depression, anxiety, and post-traumatic stress disorder.

One of the more effective psychotherapeutic methods to reduce trauma-related anxiety is called eye movement desensitization and reprocessing (EMDR). This therapy involves the patient thinking and talking about the trauma while simultaneously tracking the therapist's finger as it moves back and forth across the patient's visual field. The theory is that the side-to-side eye movement helps the brain to process the emotions associated with trauma.[15]

Treating the emotional and spiritual suffering that can be caused by trauma is more difficult. Prayer and religious faith, psychotherapy, and support groups can all be helpful.

Another way to address the emotional manifestations of trauma is by taking an energetic approach. The energetic theory of trauma is that a violent attack on your body can leave an imprint on your energy field. A patient who had experienced sexual abuse from her brother described it as feeling like "he was constantly just under my skin."

These energetic "signatures" of trauma exist outside the speech and thought centers of the brain, and thus are not able to be accessed or affected by traditional talk therapy. Energy healing is theoretically able to access and remove the energetic imprint of the trauma in a rapid, nonverbal way. One woman described feeling her "attacker's energy leaving her body" during an energy healing session, and afterwards feeling calmer and stronger emotionally.

Energy healing is a general term that describes many different techniques of accessing, channeling, balancing, and/or manipulating energy to improve health. In the conventional medical community, this is regarded with great skepticism. However, manipulation of energy (chi) for health is actually the basis of some of the more respected alternative techniques like acupuncture. And a recent study found that Tai Chi, a form of exercise designed to increase the flow of energy around the body, was beneficial in fibromyalgia.[16]

Rosalyn Bruyere, a well-known teacher of energy healing techniques, says, "The issue is in the tissue." In particular, the fascia is thought to be a storehouse for emotional energy in the body. Many myofascial release practitioners describe the release of emotions and memories related to trauma during bodywork sessions.

Finding ways to guide yourself into the relaxation response and address the long-term effects of trauma are key elements in treating in fibromyalgia, but must be individualized for each person. What gives one personal spiritual and emotional comfort might not help someone else. The same goes for inducing a relaxation response. As I said, meditation and I don't get along well, but I love yoga. Myofascial release, energy healing techniques and other ways to heal from trauma are also worth exploring.

CHAPTER RESOURCES

The Relaxation Response by Herbert Benson.

Yoga for Fibromyalgia: Move, Breathe, and Relax to Improve Your Quality of Life by Shoosh Lettick Crotzer.

Wheels of Light: Chakras, Auras, and the Healing Energy of the Body by Rosalyn Bruyere.

www.alpha-stim.com to learn more about cranial electrotherapy stimulation.

www.upledger.com for more information about craniosacral therapy.

PART III

OTHER TREATMENTS FOR FIBROMYALGIA

13

SHOULD I TAKE SUPPLEMENTS FOR FIBROMYALGIA?

One of the more common questions I am asked by patients is about which supplements they should be taking. Certainly I remember asking that same question myself when I was diagnosed, and it was very overwhelming trying to wade through all the information in books and on the Internet about supplements. At one point I was taking at least ten different supplements, which were costing me more than $300 each month and not giving me any benefit.

Unfortunately there is no good research showing that any particular vitamin, mineral, or herb is helpful in fibromyalgia (as detailed in Chapter 14). This fact has not diminished the huge array of fibromyalgia supplements promoted in books and on the Internet. It can be overwhelming when you are first diagnosed with fibromyalgia to determine what, if any, supplements you should take.

I think the key with supplements in fibromyalgia is to keep it simple. Focus on those that have some scientific support for their effectiveness, or that you personally find helpful.

Over the years I have developed a list of a few core nutrients that have been shown to support the healthy functioning of the nervous and immune system. As these are the systems of the body that are most affected by fibromyalgia, I recommend just the following few supplements to my patients, and this is what I take myself:

- Vitamin D
- B-complex vitamin
- Essential fatty acids, especially omega-3 fatty acids

Vitamin D

There is some controversy about whether people with fibromyalgia are deficient in vitamin D. Some studies have shown low blood levels of this vitamin in fibromyalgia, but some have not.[1-3] One interesting study found that people with fibromyalgia who had higher levels of anxiety and depression tended to have particularly low levels of vitamin D.[4] There is also no clear evidence that replacing vitamin D in fibromyalgia has any effect on fibromyalgia symptoms. However true vitamin D deficiency is known to cause diffuse musculoskeletal pain and weakness.[5] Typically, vitamin D is known for its role in regulating the absorption of calcium, but it has been demonstrated to have many other roles and to affect the expression of more than 200 different genes.

There has been an explosion of research into vitamin D over the last five years, and it has been found to be important in immune function and regulation of tissue growth. There are vitamin D receptors in the neurons and other brain cells.[6] Importantly, it affects how immune cells respond to bacteria and viruses. One study showed that immune cells deprived of vitamin D were not able to effectively defend against attacks from bacteria and viruses.[7]

Low vitamin D levels may also increase risk of cancer, according to one large study. However, other studies have not consistently shown this relationship.[8]

Vitamin D is a very unusual vitamin, because normally humans don't get much from their diet. It actually is produced in human skin upon exposure to sunlight. As we reduce our sun exposure due to skin cancer concerns, we are now relying more through our diet. The foods that naturally contain vitamin D include eggs and fatty fish such as salmon and mackerel. Many dairy products are now fortified with vitamin D, but in pretty low doses.

Studies show that around half of Americans are deficient in vitamin D, and that rate tends to be higher in the older population. Because it is absorbed through the skin, people with darker skin tend to absorb less, as do people who are overweight. Because most of us do not get enough sun exposure or eat enough fatty fish to get adequate intake, most experts recommend some form of supplementation for general health.

With fibromyalgia, it is particularly important that you take a vitamin D supplement, since this nutrient is so important in immune and nervous system function. I usually recommend between 2,000–5,000 IU of vitamin D daily, depending on blood levels.

Some doctors prescribe high-dose weekly vitamin D pills for patients with very low blood levels. This prescription vitamin D (ergocalciferol or D-2) is synthetic and not easily absorbed. I have not been impressed with it, as it has not produced consistent improvement in vitamin D levels in my patients. I find using the non-synthetic form of vitamin D (cholecalciferol or D-3) actually seems to work better and is available over the counter. Since vitamin D is a fat-soluble vitamin, it is best absorbed in the intestine along with fats, so I recommend taking oil-based gel capsules.

Essential fatty acids

Essential fatty acids are fats that the body does not produce itself so must be obtained from the diet. As a supplement they are best known for their cholesterol-lowering effects, but they also play an important role in the regulation of inflammation.

There are two different types of fatty acids: omega-3 and omega-6. They are both important to the healthy functioning of the human body, but tend to have opposing functions. Unfortunately, the average Western diet is much higher in the omega-6 fatty acids, and tends to be deficient in omega-3s.

This is unfortunate, because omega-3s have many important anti-inflammatory actions in the body, including the production of anti-inflammatory prostaglandins. Prostaglandins are messenger chemicals that are essential in the process of controlling inflammation. When the diet contains adequate omega-3 fatty acids, the proper balance between anti-inflammatory and pro-inflammatory prostaglandins is maintained.

But when the diet is predominantly omega-6s, the balance is skewed towards inflammation.

Scientific interest in the anti-inflammatory role of omega-3 fatty acids began after research revealed much lower rates of auto-immune and inflammatory disorders among Greenland Eskimos who consumed large amounts of omega-3s from fish.[9] This led to many studies of omega-3 supplementation in inflammatory diseases such as rheumatoid arthritis, asthma, and Crohn's disease, most of which showed at least some reduction in symptoms. In reference to rheumatoid arthritis, multiple randomized and controlled studies have shown that omega-3 supplementation results in reduced joint pain and use of anti-inflammatory drugs. Omega-3s reduced low back pain as well as ibuprofen in one study.[10]

Essential fatty acids also have important roles as components of cell walls, particularly those of the neurons, the cells of the nervous system. Increased rates of depression have been found to be associated with omega-3 deficient diets. There have been some conflicting reports, but a few studies have shown improvement of depression with omega-3 supplementation.[11-14]

I think the potential anti-inflammatory effects of omega-3 fatty acids are more than enough reason to take them as a supplement. Most supplements contain some omega-3 and some omega-6 fatty acids. It is important that you take a supplement that contains more omega-3s than omega-6s; ideally about three times more. I usually recommend a supplement of around 1,200 mg per day of omega fatty acids, so around 800mg of that should be from omega-3s. The most important omega-3 is called DHA (docosahexanoic acid), so make sure that is one of the primary ingredients listed on the nutritional breakdown.

Dietary sources of omega-3 fatty acids are mostly in oils from fatty fish such as anchovy, sardine, and mackerel. Because fatty fish can sometimes be contaminated with mercury or lead, make sure that the supplement you choose has been purified to remove these heavy metals. Flaxseed oil is the best plant source of omega-3s, but it contains much less than fish oil.

Sources of omega-6 fatty acids in the diet are from plant seed oils, such as evening primrose oils, borage seed oil, and black currant seed. The most important omega-6 to supplement is GLA (gamma-linoleic acid), so make sure this is listed on the nutrient breakdown, but it only needs to be a small amount.

There are many good supplements that contain the proper amount and types of essential fatty acids. The challenge is that many of them contain fish oil, which can taste a bit fishy and can upset the stomach and cause unpleasant "fish burps." I found one supplement when I was pregnant that contained fish oil and borage seed oil, but did not make me want to vomit. It is called Prenatal Omega Mom made by Country Life, and because it also has small amounts of peppermint and ginger oils, it has never caused me any indigestion. I continue to take it even after pregnancy.

Another trick to reduce "fish burps" is to keep your fish oil capsules in the fridge or freezer. The colder temperature keeps the oil encapsulated in the pill until after it leaves the stomach.

B vitamins

The B vitamins are water-soluble and play important roles in cell metabolism throughout the body. They are important as enzymes that help hundreds of chemical reactions in the human body, particularly in the brain and nerves. The B vitamins were once thought to be a single vitamin, but later research showed that they are in fact eight chemically distinct vitamins that often coexist in the same foods. Supplements containing all of them are generally referred to as a vitamin B complex. Because these vitamins are water-soluble, they are not stored in the body's tissues, and must constantly be replenished by diet or supplements. I recommend that all my patients with fibromyalgia take a B-complex vitamin. Some people who don't tolerate pills very well—myself included—like liquid formulations.

The most important B vitamins for the nervous system are B_6, B_{12}, and folic acid (or folate). These three vitamins aid in the production of the building blocks of protein, called amino acids that are then turned into the neurotransmitters serotonin, dopamine, and norepinephrine. You may recognize these neurotransmitters as those that are often implicated in depression. Most anti-depressants act to increase the levels of one of these neurotransmitters in the brain.

If there is a deficiency in any of these B vitamins, it can block one step in the creation of proteins and result in a buildup of potentially harmful chemicals, especially homocysteine. High levels of homocysteine are seen in some inflammatory conditions and also occur when there is a deficiency in one of these vitamins.

It is not clear if fibromyalgia is associated with low vitamin B levels. One small study found elevated homocysteine levels and decreased levels of vitamin B_{12} in the cerebrospinal fluid in fibromyalgia, which is quite intriguing but needs further study.[15]

All the B vitamins are important for nervous system health, but B_6, B_{12}, and folate also have some unique and vital functions in the body. B_6 (pyroxidine) is required for production of DNA. Inadequate amounts of B_6 result in nerve damage, confusion and skin irritation. It is widely available in our diet and is found in meats, whole grain products, vegetables, and nuts.

Vitamin B_{12} (cobalamin) is an unusual vitamin that contains the mineral cobalt in its center and is only produced in nature by tiny microorganisms like bacteria, yeasts, molds, and algae. It depends upon a second substance, called *intrinsic factor*, to be absorbed through the wall of the intestine. Without intrinsic factor, which is a unique protein made in the stomach, B_{12} cannot gain access to the rest of the body where it is needed.

Perhaps the most well-known function of B_{12} involves its role in the development of red blood cells, but it is also vital in the production and maintenance of the protective myelin sheath around nerves. B_{12} deficiency is characterized by anemia, fatigue, weakness, and neurological changes, such as numbness and tingling in the hands and feet. Additional symptoms of B_{12} deficiency include depression, confusion, and poor memory.

B_{12} is found in animal products, including fish, meat, poultry, eggs, milk, and milk products. Vegetarians in particular can suffer from low levels of B_{12} since it is generally not present in plant foods. It is found in some fortified cereal products and some nutritional yeast products.

Folate (also called folic acid) is best known for its importance in pregnancy and prevention of birth defects. However, it plays a vital role in the production of new cells, because it is needed to make DNA and RNA, the genetic material inside cells. It is also needed in order to make red blood cells. Folate deficiency can result in anemia, depression, peripheral neuropathy, forgetfulness, confusion, insomnia, and weakness.

There has been a great deal of research into a connection between low folate levels and depression. About one third of patients with depression also have a folate deficiency.[16]

Folate is found in the diet in leafy green vegetables (like spinach and turnip greens), citrus fruits, beans, and peas. Dietary supplements generally contain folate in the synthetic form of folic acid. Both folate from food and folic acid from supplements are absorbed through the intestines, and then have to go through four separate biochemical transformations to become L-methylfolate, the form that is actually useable by the body.

Some people have a mildly dysfunctional form of one enzyme necessary to change folic acid into L-methylfolate, and interestingly, tend to have higher rates of depression. One study found that 70 percent of depressed patients had the gene for this dysfunctional enzyme.[17]

In addition to insufficient dietary intake or difficulty processing folate into a useable form, there are other factors that can influence levels in the body. Certain medication such as anticonvulsants (lamotrignine and valproate), methotrexate, metformin, and oral contraceptives can lower folate levels. Alcohol, smoking, and pregnancy can also deplete the body of folate.

Prescription supplements

Most people, with or without fibromyalgia, would benefit from taking a B-complex vitamin daily. However, in some people with fibromyalgia I do recommend taking prescription B-vitamin supplements, which are also called "medical foods."

In particular, I prescribe L-methylfolate (Deplin) for my patients with ongoing depression even while on an anti-depressant. L-methylfolate is the active form of folate that is easily utilized by the brain to make neurotransmitters, bypassing the step that requires the enzyme that may be deficient in some people. Several studies have shown some improvement in depression with L-methylfolate alone, or when added to other antidepressants.[18-20] Some of my patients have noticed no benefit from Deplin, but for others it has seemed to improve their depression.

For fibromyalgia patients with neuropathy (nerve damage resulting in tingling, numbness, and pain), I will prescribe a different prescription B vitamin called Metanx. In addition to L-methylfolate, it contains the most active forms of B_6 (pyridoxal 5'-phosphate) and B_{12} (methylcobalamin). This supplement has shown reduced pain in diabetic neuropathy in a few small studies, but no study has been done in fibromyalgia.[21] The central sensitization of the nervous system in fibromyalgia seems to respond to the same type of pharmaceutical medications as diabetic neuropathy, so it stands to reason that fibromyalgia patients might get benefit from Metanx as well. But certainly more research needs to be done on this supplement before it can be recommended for all patients with fibromyalgia.

Unfortunately, because Deplin and Metanx are considered medical foods, most insurance plans will not pay for them, and they cost about $70–80 for a month's supply. However, if you have fibromyalgia plus either depression or neuropathy, these prescription vitamin B supplements might be worth a try.

CHAPTER RESOURCES

Good, reliable vitamin information can be found at the website for the NIH Office of Dietary supplements at www.dietarysupplements.info. nih.gov/Health_Information/Vitamin_and_Mineral_Supplement_Fact_Sheets.aspx.

www.deplin.com

www.metanx.com

14

EFFECTIVE ALTERNATIVE THERAPIES—WHAT HELPS AND WHAT DOESN'T

This may be most useful and cost-effective section in this book. After my fibromyalgia diagnosis, I pretty quickly realized that conventional Western medicine had little to offer me. I was desperate and spent hours combing the Internet to find something, anything that could help me. The sheer volume of alternative theories and fibromyalgia treatments promoted on the Internet promising to cure all my ills was completely overwhelming. I ended up trying many of them, and spent literally thousands of wasted dollars on various ineffective supplements, diets, and treatments.

One patient told me she spent more than $50,000 over seven years on various alternative treatments, and that none had really helped her. But feelings of desperation lead people into the uncharted waters of alternative medicine.

I ready every book I could find about fibromyalgia, and just became more confused. The best-selling book, *From Fatigued to Fantastic*, described a dizzying array of supplements and treatment suggestions for fibromyalgia. I felt like I had to be my own doctor, and try to figure out my own treatment plan based on conflicting theories and approaches.

There are some alternative therapies that are very helpful in fibromyalgia. The challenge is that there are a lot of snake-oil salesman out there trying to sell supplements and treatments that are useless. How do we figure out which alternative treatments might actually help? The only way is to do it scientifically and look at the research.

This chapter summarizes the research on various alternative treatments for fibromyalgia, and also includes some of my personal and clinical experience. Hopefully this chapter will save you some time, money, and frustration.

First a note about interpreting terms used in medical research. The most ideal study design that gathers the most reliable and useful data is called a randomized, controlled, double-blind study. What do these terms mean?

- **Controlled**: Patients are divided into two groups, one that gets a treatment, and one that gets a placebo (a fake treatment). With medications, a placebo is usually a sugar pill.

- **Randomized**: Patients are put randomly into each group.

- **Double blind**: Both patients and researchers don't know which treatment each study participant is getting.

The closer a study is to this model, the higher its quality, meaning that the results are unlikely to be due to placebo effect or other factors that can skew results.

As you can imagine, this ideal type of study is not always possible, but other study designs provide weaker evidence. For example, with certain treatments, such as fasting, you cannot blind the patient as they can certainly tell if they are eating or not. If there is no control group in a study, it is harder to tell if any study findings are due to the placebo effect or to the treatment being tested.

A placebo effect occurs when a treatment or medication with no therapeutic value (a placebo) is administered to a patient and the patient's symptoms improve. The patient believes and expects that the treatment is going to work, and it does in some measure, whether in reality or perception. The goal of research is to measure the efficacy of the administered treatment beyond any placebo effect.

I have scoured the published medical literature to find studies that address some of the most commonly used treatments in fibromyalgia.

Unfortunately, not every treatment or supplement that you might hear about has been analyzed in a formal, published study. Some treatments have no published evidence to evaluate. I have added some information about effective treatments from my personal and clinical experience with fibromyalgia patients, but primarily the focus of this chapter is on those alternative treatments that have been studied for fibromyalgia.

Alternative medicine therapies

Cleansing and detoxifying: This includes various fasting techniques, colonics, and enemas, in addition to herbal compounds that purport to "rid your body of toxins." After devoting about six months of my life and thousands of dollars to these techniques, I found no benefit and actually felt worse.

However, one small study on an eight-day supervised fasting regimen did find a small improvement in pain in fibromyalgia, however there was no control group. As I describe elsewhere, I think improvements seen with fasting are due to avoidance of allergens, not due to fasting itself or to any detoxifying action.[1]

Acupuncture: This is a very common alternative medicine technique used by fibromyalgia patients. One survey found that almost one quarter of fibromyalgia patients had tried acupuncture.[2] Certainly, it causes no harm, and some of my patients get some improvement with acupuncture. Overall the evidence is fairly weak that acupuncture helps in fibromyalgia. In two recent high-quality, randomized, controlled trials, acupuncture was no better than control interventions (sham acupuncture) for fibromyalgia. However, some researchers feel this might be explained by the fact that "sham" acupuncture' is so similar to acupuncture that patients are actually getting benefits from that as well.[3]

Certainly, acupuncture is very safe and may be worth a try if you can afford it. I personally did not get much benefit from it for my fibromyalgia symptoms, but it helped a lot with my morning sickness in pregnancy.

Magnets: One small study showed improvement in pain and sleep in fibromyalgia patients using magnets. But a larger six-month study of sleeping on magnetic pads in fibromyalgia found no difference in symptoms sleeping on a non-magnetic pad compared to a placebo pad.[4, 5]

Microcurrent therapy: This treatment involves the application of very small amounts of electric current to the skin, which is thought to penetrate the soft tissue and stimulate healing. This low dose electrical current is theoretically similar to the electrical signal cells use to communicate with each other in the body, and can therefore promote the natural electrical cellular reactions in the healing process. The current can be applied to the skin either by pads or through special conducting gloves that the therapist wears and places on the client's body.

One uncontrolled study (meaning no placebo group) showed improved pain in fibromyalgia patients after microcurrent therapy, in addition to reduced levels of inflammatory chemicals in the blood stream.[6] I have not tried this therapy myself, but a few of my patients have had some success with it in healing nagging soft-tissue injuries. However, it is expensive (around $100 per session), and generally not covered by insurance.

Cold laser therapy: This works on similar principles to microcurrent therapy, but instead of electricity it uses a concentrated light beam. The type of laser used is called a "cold" laser, because it is a very low dose of light that does not burn the tissue. The theory is that low doses of light applied to soft tissue will stimulate accelerated healing at the cellular level. Two small studies showed some mild improvement in fibromyalgia pain with laser therapy applied for three minutes at each tender point for two weeks.[7, 8]

There is some science supporting the use of lasers in other conditions. Cold laser treatment has been shown to speed up wound healing of the skin, and to reduce pain in tennis elbow.[9-11] In the lab, tissue cells such as fibroblasts that are exposed to lasers multiply faster and secrete more collagen and growth factors, all of which are very important in the healing process.[12, 13]

As described earlier, there is some evidence that fibroblasts are not functioning normally in fibromyalgia. It is possible that laser therapy could improve fibroblast healing and reduce pain in fibromyalgia. However, one large study using laser therapy for myofascial pain of the neck and shoulders did not show any benefit compared to placebo.[14] Clearly, more research needs to be done before we can determine the effectiveness of laser therapy in fibromyalgia.

Interestingly, a technique similar to cold laser therapy that uses infra-red (or near-infrared light) is being explored by NASA. Infrared light is not visible to the human eye, but can be seen by night-vision goggles. The red and infrared light emitted from light-emitting diodes (LEDs) has been shown in several NASA and military experiments to improve tissue heal-ing.[15] This therapy has not been tested in fibromyalgia, however. LEDs are much cheaper and easier to use than low-level laser therapy, so if shown to be effective in fibromyalgia could be easily used at home. Laser therapy has to be administered in a health care setting, if done incorrectly can be dangerous, and is quite expensive.

Bodywork: Manual therapy can be helpful in fibromyalgia, but it very much depends on the type of therapy. Most patients tell me that massage feels good during a session, but the effects only last a few hours. There are a wide variety of massage techniques, however, and some may be more helpful than others.

As far as typical Swedish massage, I did not find it helpful. It seemed to make me more achy and sore for a few days. But one study did find that fibromyalgia patients that received massage twice weekly for five weeks, experienced decreased pain and had fewer tender points.[16] See Chapter 11 for more explanation on manual therapy in fibromyalgia.

I found that myofascial release gave me longer lasting pain relief than a massage. No direct studies of this therapy in fibromyalgia have yet been published. A study of connective tissue massage in fibromyalgia, a tech-nique with some similarities to myofascial release, found reduced pain, improved depression and quality of life compared to a control group.[17]

Another study showed benefits from an osteopathic manipula-tive treatment (OMT) that incorporated some myofascial release techniques.[18]

Vitamins, minerals, and supplements: There is no convincing evidence for any particular supplement in fibromyalgia, in part because not that many studies have been performed. There are a few supplements that I recommend for my patients, but even those are based mostly on theoretical effectiveness rather than research evidence (see Chapter 13).

Guaifenesin: This is an over-the-counter expectorant medicine that has been proposed as a treatment for fibromyalgia. The theory behind use of this medication is that it can reduce pain by removing irritating calcium phosphate deposits from the tissue. Although it is the subject of a popular book (*What Your Doctor May Not Tell You About Fibromyalgia: The Revolutionary Treatment That Can Reverse the Disease*) which has a devoted internet following, guaifenesin was found to be no more effective than placebo in a well-designed study 12-month study.[19] There is also no evidence supporting the theory that calcium tissue deposits are behind the muscle pain in fibromyalgia.

S-adenosyl methionine (SAMe): This supplement has been shown in two small studies to have some beneficial effects on some measures of mood and pain in fibromyalgia, but not on others. SAMe contains the amino acid methionine, and is involved in many different synthetic pathways in the body, including production of other amino acids, proteins, and neurotransmitters. It is possible that it might help in fibromyalgia as a supplement because amino acids can stimulate growth hormone release. Larger studies would need to be done to determine its true effectiveness in fibromyalgia. Unfortunately, combining SAMe with antidepressants carries a risk of causing serotonin syndrome, a potentially deadly excess of serotonin in the brain.[20, 21]

Magnesium/Malic acid: Researchers at the University of Texas studied Super Malic (magnesium 50mg and malic acid 200mg per tablet) in a small randomized controlled trial on 24 fibromyalgia patients, and found it to be no better than placebo. After the placebo-controlled stage of the study there was an open-label trial, meaning everyone in the study knew they were taking Super Malic. They also increased the dose in this part of the study. There was some symptom improvement in the latter half of the study, but it is impossible to know if this improvement was due to the placebo effect or not.[22]

Intravenous micronutrient therapy (Myer's cocktail): This is a popular naturopathic treatment for fibromyalgia and chronic fatigue, and is an intravenous infusion of magnesium, calcium, vitamin C and B vitamins. A well-designed study found no difference between eight weeks of weekly Myer's cocktail infusions versus placebo.[23]

D-Ribose: This is a simple carbohydrate (sugar) that is thought to be helpful in increasing energy production in muscle cells. A small study of patients, some with chronic fatigue syndrome and some with fibromyalgia, showed significant improvement in energy, sleep, mental clarity, and well-being. This study was done by Dr. Jacob Teitelbaum, who describes it in further detail in his book, *From Fatigued to Fantastic*. Unfortunately, the study had no placebo group, and was "open-label," meaning patients knew what they were taking, so it is hard to know if the positive effects were due to the treatment or due to placebo effect.[24]

Hormones

Dehydroepiandrosterone (DHEA): This is a steroid hormone released from the adrenal glands that is turned into estrogens and testosterone. DHEA supplementation did not improve pain, mood, or fatigue in fibromyalgia in a randomized controlled trial.[25] Many naturopaths will treat fatigue with different steroid supplementation, such as hydrocortisone. While no studies have specifically assessed hydrocortisone in fibromyalgia, the philosophy behind using it does not make much sense to me. As you know, the problem in fibromyalgia is that the stress response system is overactive, and thus the adrenal glands are constantly pouring out stress hormones. Adding extra artificial stress hormones to the mix doesn't seem likely to improve this situation.

Growth hormone: This hormone is secreted by the pituitary gland in the brain, and is important for healthy tissue growth and repair. As you have read, most people with fibromyalgia do not make enough of this hormone. Dr. Rob Bennett and his coworkers treated a group of fibromyalgia patients with daily injections of growth hormone for nine months, and found fibromyalgia symptom improvement. After discontinuing the growth hormone injections, patients experienced a worsening of symptoms.[26] Another study found a 60 percent reduction in pain in fibromyalgia patients with growth hormone injections.[27]

However, growth hormone injections are very expensive and carry an increased risk of cancer (since growth hormone can stimulate growth of abnormal tissue as well), making this not a viable treatment option for fibromyalgia. A safer way to increase growth hormone levels in fibromyalgia is to increase deep sleep. There is a potential new treatment option that increases deep sleep and growth hormone in fibromyalgia that is discussed in detail in Chapter 10.

Thyroid hormone: Some alternative practitioners advocate for supplementing this hormone in fibromyalgia, even if lab tests show the thyroid functioning normally. Most studies measuring thyroid hormone tests have found them to be consistently normal in fibromyalgia. Lab tests measure the levels of thyroid stimulating hormone (TSH) released from the brain and the two different forms of thyroid hormone that circulate in the body (T3 and T4).

One theory is that although the thyroid is functioning normally in fibromyalgia, perhaps the cells of the body are not absorbing and utilizing the thyroid hormone correctly. This could result in symptoms of underactive thyroid and explain the fatigue and weakness that are seen in fibromyalgia. Some very vocal practitioners claim that all of the symptoms of fibromyalgia are actually due to thyroid hormone issues, and can be eliminated by hormone supplementation.

There is not much evidence to support the use of thyroid supplements in fibromyalgia, but to be fair this has not been studied in-depth due to concerns about dangerous side effects. A few studies have shown higher than normal levels of antibodies against thyroid tissue in subjects with fibromyalgia, but the significance of these antibodies are not clear, as they also appear in some healthy people.[28, 29]

Two small studies found improvement in fibromyalgia symptoms in people taking thyroid supplements, but unfortunately these were not high quality studies and further research in this area is lacking.[30, 31]

This is a very controversial topic about which conventional medicine and naturopathic medicine generally disagree. Most Western medical doctors treat based on the lab tests exclusively, and are concerned about the dangers of excess thyroid hormone. Naturopathic doctors try to treat based on patient symptoms more than the lab tests.

The jury is still out about thyroid hormone supplementation in fibromyalgia. In my clinical practice, I have not had a single patient tell me they really noticed much difference when taking thyroid supplements, except for those that had abnormal lab tests indicating hypothyroidism. Unfortunately, several of my patients developed heart problems while taking thyroid supplements prescribed by a naturopath. The potential risks of excess thyroid hormone are very serious, and include hyperthyroidism, abnormal heart rhythms and osteoporosis.

Dietary changes: Two small studies on raw food vegetarian diets (primarily fruits, vegetables and nuts) in fibromyalgia did show improvement in stiffness, pain, and quality of life. These improvements rapidly disappeared after returning to regular diet.[32, 33] As you can imagine, with diet studies it is impossible to "blind" the participants, because people know what they are eating. There may be a significant placebo effect in diet studies. It is also possible that a raw food or vegan diet is so different from the average American's diet that it effectively eliminates all allergens. This might explain the improvements seen in these studies.

Another study using ELISA/ACT blood testing to identify allergies noted marked improvement in fibromyalgia symptoms upon dietary changes to avoid the allergens, although there was no control group.[34] This is the same testing that I used (and is described in detail in Chapter 6). To get the most benefit from dietary changes they need to be individualized to each person's intolerances and allergies to various foods.

Exercise: There have been more than 75 studies to date on exercise in fibromyalgia, and almost all of them show that fibromyalgia patients get benefits from exercise, including decreased pain and improved quality of life (for more details see Chapter 9). Benefits are seen with all types of exercise, including aerobic, strength, and flexibility training. For the most part, patients with fibromyalgia tolerate exercise well, as long as it is of low to moderate intensity. Only one study of high-intensity strength training caused fibromyalgia symptoms to worsen.[35]

Aerobic exercise in pools shows additional benefits for fibromyalgia, with greater improvements in mood and sleep compared to land aerobics. Exercising in warm water is particularly helpful, probably because the warmth eases muscle spasm and stiffness. Very low-impact exercise like yoga tend to be helpful and well tolerated.[36] A recent study in the New England Journal of Medicine found that Tai Chi, an ancient Chinese martial art, reduced fibromyalgia symptoms. Tai Chi is a unique combination of gentle movement, deep breathing and relaxation techniques. [37]

The following table (next page) summarizes the research on the effectiveness of alternative therapies and ranks the quality of the evidence as high, medium, or low:

Treatment	Helpful or not in fibromyalgia?	Quality of evidence
Guaifenesin	not helpful	high
IV micronutrient therapy (Myer's cocktail)	not helpful	high
DHEA	not helpful	high
Growth hormone	helpful, but risky	high
Magnet therapy	not helpful	high
Exercise	helpful	high
Laser therapy	helpful	medium
Manual therapy	helpful	medium
SAMe	helpful	medium
IV lidocaine	helpful , but risky	medium
Fasting/Cleansing	possibly helpful	low
D-ribose	possibly helpful	low
Raw food/vegetarian diet	possibly helpful	low
Diet changes based on allergy testing	helpful	low
Microcurrent therapy	helpful	low
Magnesium/malic acid	possibly helpful	low
Thyroid hormone	possibly helpful	low

15

PRESCRIPTION MEDICATIONS
THAT CAN HELP

The interest of pharmaceutical companies in fibromyalgia began in earnest in 2002, when central sensitization was finally documented in fibromyalgia. Once there was a definite target—increased pain processing in the spinal cord and brain—there was an explosion of funding in the pharmaceutical industry for fibromyalgia treatments.

It wasn't until 2008 that a medication was finally granted approval by the U.S. Food and Drug Administration (FDA) for use in fibromyalgia. The first was duloxetine (Cymbalta), followed by pregabalin (Lyrica) and milnacipran (Savella). These three are currently the only FDA-approved medications for use in fibromyalgia, but there are many other medications that are frequently prescribed for this condition. Sodium oxybate is a very exciting new sleep medication for fibromyalgia that is currently being evaluated by the FDA.

There are some small studies supporting the use of other medications in fibromyalgia, but since these are older medicines whose patent has expired, there is no pharmaceutical industry sponsored research for these medications. It takes a great deal of money and research to get enough evidence to get an FDA-approval for a medication in a specific disease (also called an indication). Unless a drug company is sponsoring the trials, it is very rare for an older, generic medication to get FDA-approval for a new indication.

However once a drug has been FDA-approved for use in any condition, it can legally be prescribed for other conditions in what is called "off-label" prescribing. Many health insurances will only pay for a medication that has been FDA-approved for the condition for which it was prescribed—unless of course that medicine is generic and dirt cheap, and then often the insurance will pay for it. Thus, much less research is being done on older medications commonly used in fibromyalgia.

In this chapter, I discuss all the medications currently being used to treat fibromyalgia. The most commonly prescribed medications for fibromyalgia are anti-depressants and anti-convulsants, but there are many others being used, including some experimental and controversial drugs. I review the pros and cons of the variety of medications used based on available research studies and my clinical experience with these medicines.

Anti-convulsants (Lyrica and Neurontin): These were originally developed as anti-seizure medications, but were found not to be very effective in preventing seizures. Instead they were found to reduce some types of pain, especially neuropathic pain (pain from damaged or inflamed nerves). They reduce nerve pain by decreasing the speed and intensity of pain signals coming into the spinal cord.

Both pregabalin (Lyrica) and gabapentin (Neurontin) have been have been found in multiple studies to reduce pain in fibromyalgia. Neurontin is an older generic medication that is similar to Lyrica, but is not FDA-approved in fibromyalgia. However, it has many of the same benefits and is cheaper, so it is frequently used in treating fibromyalgia. In addition to pain reduction, there is some evidence that these medications may help fatigue and improve sleep. One study found that treatment with Lyrica actually increased the amount and duration of deep sleep.[1]

Unfortunately, both these medications have a high frequency of side effects, including weight gain, water retention, and dizziness. In clinical trials, between 19–33 percent of patients on Lyrica stopped treatment due to side effects.[2] Side effects can be reduced by starting doses low and increasing them slowly.

In my practice, many patients don't tolerate these medications very well, which limits their usefulness. Some patients do get significant improvement with these drugs. I estimate that of every 10 people for whom I prescribe Lyrica, only about two patients will have enough improvement in pain to continue taking the medicine. The majority stop due to intolerable side effects like feeling drunk or dizzy, or rapid weight gain and swelling due to water retention. Fortunately, all these side effects are reversible after stopping the medication. Neurontin does seem to be better tolerated, although can have many of the same problems.

Serotonin and Norepinephrine Reuptake Inhibitors (SNRIs) (Cymbalta, Savella and Effexor): These antidepressants can reduce pain in addition to improving mood in fibromyalgia. This type of medication increases the levels of serotonin and norepinepephrine in the brain, which helps to filter out pain signals. Interestingly, antidepressants that affect only serotonin, such as fluoxetine (Prozac) have not been shown to reduce pain in fibromyalgia. Only those antidepressants that affect both neurotransmitters (serotonin and norepinephrine) have shown any benefit for pain in fibromyalgia. Both duloxetine (Cymbalta) and milnacipran (Savella) are FDA-approved for fibromyalgia. A similar older medication venlafaxine (Effexor) is not quite as effective but is much cheaper.[3]

The SNRIs are generally well-tolerated, the most common side effects are nausea, excess sweating, and increased heart rate. Some of my patients have experienced 30–40 percent reduction in their pain on this type of medicine, but usually the benefits are much milder.

Tricyclic antidepressants (amitriptyline, nortriptyline): These older medications have mild effects on serotonin and norepinephrine levels in the brain. They can be modestly helpful in fibromyalgia, but they also affect many other chemicals in the brain and tend to have a lot of side effects. One of the major side effects is sleepiness, so they are often used at night and can be effective for insomnia.[4] However, they often cause grogginess in the morning.

I never found any personal benefit from any of these medications, and they all made me feel quite "hung over" and foggy the next day. However, for some of my patients they are helpful with sleep, and they are inexpensive.

Dopamine agonists (Requip, Mirapex, Sinemet): Dopamine is another neurotransmitter (chemical messenger in the brain). Dopamine-agonist medications act by stimulating dopamine receptors in the brain. The rationale for using them in fibromyalgia is that increased dopamine activity may be able to calm the fight-or-flight nervous system activity that interferes with sleep in fibromyalgia. A randomized controlled double-blind study found treatment with pramipexole (Mirapex) resulted in some improvement in pain, fatigue, and functioning in fibromyalgia.[5] Side effects in the treatment group included weight loss, nausea, and anxiety. This type of medicine is also used to treat restless legs syndrome, and I find my patients with this condition along with fibromyalgia tend to get the most benefit from this type of medicine.

The author of the Mirapex study theorizes that short-term exposure to high doses of dopamine might be able to "reset" the balance in the auto-pilot nervous system and reverse the fight-or-flight dominance. More research needs to be done but there may be some potential in this treatment. Serious side effects can develop from exposure to high doses of dopamine, however. The most concerning side effect seen is the sudden onset of an impulse control disorder, like gambling, excessive shopping, or hypersexuality. One of my patients began compulsively collecting rocks, and another couldn't stop ordering from TV shopping programs. I think these side effects will limit the practical usefulness of these medications in fibromyalgia.

Anti-inflammatories: This group of medications includes steroids such as prednisone, and non-steroidal anti-inflammatories (NSAIDS) like ibuprofen. No improvements in fibromyalgia symptoms were reported with prednisone 15 mg per day for two weeks, or with the NSAID medications ibuprofen and naproxen.[6-8] Generally these medications are not very helpful with fibromyalgia muscle pain, although sometimes they do help with pain from osteoarthritis.

Oral NSAIDS also can increase risk of bleeding ulcers. Some new prescription topical NSAIDS have recently come on the market in the United States. These include the Flector patch, Voltaren gel, and Pennsaid liquid.

These topical medications have much lower absorption into the bloodstream, so cause fewer side effects and seem to work better for muscle pain. I personally have found Voltaren gel to be really helpful in reducing pain from overuse injuries like tendinitis or plantar fasciitis.

Muscle relaxants (Soma, Zanaflex, Robaxin, Skelaxin, Flexeril): These medications are frequently prescribed for fibromyalgia, with mixed results. My patients tend to have the most benefit from carisoprodol (Soma) and cyclobenzaprine (Flexeril). I rarely prescribe muscle relaxants in my practice because they just don't seem to help that much in fibromyalgia.

Muscle relaxants act on the brain to reduce signals to the muscles, which seems like it should really help with the tense muscles of fibromyalgia. However, the unique tension of fibromyalgia muscles does not seem to respond well to muscle relaxants. Since these drugs act on the brain, they do have frequent side effects of drowsiness and dizziness. They are often prescribed to take at bedtime, and can be helpful with sleep.

The best-studied muscle relaxant is cyclobenzaprine, which was one of the first medications to show any benefit in fibromyalgia. Studies consistently show mild improvements seen in sleep and pain.[9] Interestingly, cyclobenzaprine is chemically related to the tricyclic antidepressants, which may explain some of its effectiveness.

The other muscle relaxant my patients tend to find helpful is carisoprodol. A small study also showed that it helped with fibromyalgia symptoms.[10] Unfortunately, this medication can lead to dependence and addiction, similar to benzodiazepines and opiates. If stopped suddenly withdrawal symptoms may occur, and it can be very dangerous, even deadly, when taken with other sedative medications. These concerns limit its usefulness, and many doctors refuse to prescribe it. Several European countries have recently taken carisoprodol off the market due to safety concerns and abuse potential.

Medical marijuana: I am asked at least once a day by patients if marijuana might help with fibromyalgia symptoms. This is a hard question to answer, since we really have a lack of scientific information to help us decide if it is useful. Marijuana (also called cannabis) is only legalized for medical use in 14 U.S. states, and is a very controversial subject. I happen to practice medicine in Oregon, a state that has a large amount of medical marijuana usage.

Some of my patients who have tried it tell me they found it helpful, while others have not—just like any other medication. Several have told me that brewing the leaves as a tea and drinking it before bed seems to result in improved sleep quality.

Unfortunately there have been zero studies looking at marijuana in fibromyalgia. There have only been a handful of studies in other painful conditions. In one recent study, pain from neuropathy (damaged nerves) was reduced by smoking marijuana.[11]

An oral medication that activates some of the same receptors in the brain as marijuana, nabilone, has been studied in fibromyalgia. This synthetic oral cannabinoid is used primarily as an anti-nausea agent during chemotherapy. One small study reported a reduction in fibromyalgia pain with use of nabilone.[12]

Another study found that fibromyalgia subjects reported improved quality of sleep and feeling more rested in the morning when taking nabilone.[13] Unfortunately, no measurements of sleep stages or quality were done as part of this study, as it was simply based on patients' self-report of sleep quality. One study from 1975 did find that use of marijuana increased time spent in deeper stages of sleep for healthy people, but this has not been confirmed in fibromyalgia.[14]

More research needs to be done on the use of marijuana as a medicine for fibromyalgia. Nabilone is quite expensive, and there is probably not enough data at this point to justify its use, but this is an area of active research.

Opiates (morphine, codeine, hydrocodone, oxycodone, methadone, fentanyl, hydromorphone): The use of opiate-based pain medications in fibromyalgia is controversial, primarily because of the lack of data supporting their effectiveness and the high risk for the abuse and addiction. However they are frequently prescribed - one study found that 25% fibromyalgia patients receive one of these medications.[15]

Opiates (also called opioids) are derived from the poppy plant, and act in the body at certain receptors in the brain and spinal cord to reduce pain. These receptors, called opiate receptors, also bind endorphins, the body's natural pain-relieving chemicals.

There is very little supporting evidence for long-term opiate use in fibromyalgia, but frankly not that many studies have been done.[16] Long-term opiate use for any reason tends to result in worsened functional outcomes; more depression, weight gain, and disability.[17] In addition, when taken chronically, opiates can actually increase sensitivity to pain, a phenomenon called opiate-induced hyperalgesia.

In fibromyalgia, there is some evidence that opiates used chronically might actually increase the central sensitization that is already part of the condition.[18] Clinically, opiates don't seem to work that well for fibromyalgia pain, and studies have shown that too. One study found that IV morphine did not result in any noticeable reduction in fibromyalgia pain.[19]

Another study found that people with fibromyalgia have fewer opiate receptors in their brain. This means there would be fewer places for opiate medicines to bind in the brain, and thus fewer pain-relieving effects.[20] Finally, sleep studies show that opiate-based pain medications reduce deep sleep, and, as you can imagine, that effect could make symptoms even worse in fibromyalgia.[21]

The only analgesic (pain-reliever) that has evidence of effectiveness in fibromyalgia is tramadol (Ultram).[22, 23] This is a unique medication that acts partly like an opiate pain killer but also increases levels of serotonin and norepinephrine in the brain, which increases the brain's ability to filter out pain signals.

Tramadol is less addictive with a lower abuse potential than other opiates, and is not currently treated as a controlled substance. However, there have been reports of abuse and withdrawal symptoms upon discontinuation, and in the future it may be treated more like other opiate pain medicines. Because this medication increases serotonin levels in the brain, it can be dangerous to combine with other medications that also increase serotonin levels like anti-depressants. There is a risk of developing serotonin syndrome—a relatively rare condition of excess serotonin in the brain that can be life threatening. The symptoms of this syndrome can develop rapidly, and may include confusion, fast heart rate, hallucinations, increased body temperature, and even seizures. The potential risk of serotonin syndrome unfortunately limits the use of tramadol in fibromyalgia patients who are already taking antidepressants.

In my practice, I have found that small amounts of low-dose opiates used occasionally during pain crises can be helpful. For the most part, my fibromyalgia patients seem to do better overall when not taking opiates daily. Since opiates are not very effective in fibromyalgia and also interfere with deep sleep it makes sense to avoid them as much as possible and use only short-term for severe pain flares.

Naltrexone: Interestingly, while opiate medications have not shown much benefit in fibromyalgia, an opiate-blocking medication called naltrexone may be helpful. Naltrexone acts to block opiate receptors in the brain and spinal cord, but does not activate the receptor itself. You can think of it as a key that fits into the lock of a door, but does not open the door. This is the opposite of what opiates like morphine do; they fit in the lock and swing the door wide open, activating the opiate receptor. Naltrexone is most commonly used in addiction treatment for both alcoholism and opiate addiction. It blocks the opiate receptors so other opiates and chemicals can't activate them.

However, low-dose naltrexone was found to reduce pain in fibromyalgia in one small study. This was a pilot study on 10 women who did not know what medication they were taking. For the first two weeks, all the women took a placebo pill. Then they took the naltrexone for eight weeks, then nothing for two weeks. During the placebo period, pain scores reduced by two percent. During the drug period, pain scores reduced by 33 percent. Most importantly, during the drug period, experimental tests of the reactivity of the nervous system found decreased response of the nervous system to mechanical pain and heat pain. So in addition to feeling better on naltrexone, these patients were actually able to tolerate more pressure and more heat before it became painful, which means that the central sensitization was actually reduced.[24]

These results are surprising, because as an opiate-blocker, you would expect naltrexone to cause increased pain and less tolerance to painful stimuli. It turns out that the effect of naltrexone on pain may not involve the opiate receptors at all. Naltrexone also blocks receptors on glial cells, the support cells surrounding the neurons of the spinal cord that play a huge role in development of spinal cord reactivity.[25] In rats that have had spinal cord hyper-reactivity induced by nerve injury, naltrexone results in less sensitivity to pain and less amplification of pain signals in the spinal cord.

A larger study on naltrexone in fibromyalgia is currently ongoing at Stanford University, sponsored by the American Fibromyalgia Syndrome Association.

Intravenous (IV) lidocaine: Lidocaine is a common local anesthetic (numbing) agent that is used in surgery and dental procedures. It causes a slowing of electrical signals in the nerves, and this results in reduced pain sensation. Every paramedic and physician is familiar with the other common use of lidocaine: injected intravenously in emergencies, it can slow down dangerously fast heart rates such as ventricular fibrillation. When injected into the bloodstream, lidocaine slows the heart rate because it slows down electrical signals in the heart.

The mechanism by which IV lidocaine might reduce pain in fibromyalgia is not certain. Some researchers think it is due to a direct effect on the spinal cord. However others, myself included, think that lidocaine could reduce pain by numbing the irritated peripheral nerves in the fascia in fibromyalgia. One study found that IV lidocaine reduced pain in fibromyalgia much more then IV morphine did.[19] A few of my patients that have received lidocaine infusions at naturopathic clinics tell me they found it very helpful in reducing their pain for about a week. Two small studies have also found significant, but temporary, reduction in pain in fibromyalgia.[26, 27]

There are some concerns about the safety of this therapy. Since IV lidocaine also affects the heart, it can have very serious cardiac side effects. One study looking at the safety of IV lidocaine infusions found that out of 106 fibromyalgia patients given IV lidocaine, 42 reported minor side effects and two had major cardiac side effects. The cardiac side effects included one case of supraventricular tachycardia (abnormal heart rate) and one case of pulmonary edema (fluid in the lungs), both requiring treatment. In addition, 17 people had episodes of low blood pressure while getting the infusion, which required slowing or stopping of the infusion.

Because of the potential for lidocaine to cause cardiac side effects, the authors of the safety study recommended continuous monitoring of heart rhythm and pulse while undergoing this therapy, and that it be done only in medical settings equipped to deal with emergencies.[28] As you can imagine, that means it can be quite expensive. It is also not covered by most insurance. At this point, the potential risks of this therapy outweigh the temporary benefits. If you do choose to try this type of therapy, make sure you understand the risks and have it performed in a monitored, medical setting.

Sleep medications (Ambien, Lunesta, Sonata, Ativan, Xanax, Klonopin, Valium): All of these sleep medications can help you to fall asleep faster but do not increase deep-sleep time. They increase sleep quantity, but not quality, and none of them have shown any benefit in reducing fibromyalgia symptoms of pain or fatigue.[29-31] What these medications can treat is insomnia (the inability to fall asleep), and some bad sleep is better than no sleep at all.

The anti-anxiety medications called benzodiazepines—which includes alprazolam (Xanax) and diazepam (Valium)—are used to treat insomnia, anxiety, and restless leg symptoms. The benzodiazepines can be addictive, and if stopped suddenly can have severe withdrawal reaction. They can also be deadly when combined with other sedatives or opiate pain medications. So I prescribe these very carefully, and usually only to people with severe restless legs symptoms.

Other sleeping medications like zolpidem (Ambien), zopiclone (Lunesta), and zaleplon (Sonata) are safer and less addictive. I frequently prescribe them to treat insomnia.

A new medication that increases deep sleep is currently awaiting FDA-approval for use in fibromyalgia based on some very positive initial studies. Sodium oxybate (Xyrem) is known for its sedative effects and for its ability to induce deep restorative sleep.[32,33] This is a somewhat controversial medication, as detailed in Chapter 10.

Stimulant medications (Adderall, Ritalin, Provigil, Nuvigil): Some patients benefit from the use of stimulant medications to treat the fatigue and brain fog associated with fibromyalgia. I tend to avoid prescribing the stimulant medications that are derived from amphetamines (Adderall and Ritalin) due to the risk of addiction and cardiac problems. A newer medication, modafinil (Provigil), is not an amphetamine, but promotes alertness by stimulating the part of the brain that controls wakefulness. It is much safer than the amphetamine-derived medications and less addictive. Provigil, and a related medication called Nuvigil, are commonly used to treat the sleepiness of narcolepsy and other sleep conditions. I have had some fibromyalgia patients find they reduce fatigue and help them to be more functional during the day. Several case reports have been published about positive effects in fibromyalgia, but no large clinical trials have been performed.[34, 35] Unfortunately, both Provigil and Nuvigil are quite expensive and not usually covered by insurance to treat fibromyalgia-related fatigue.

CHAPTER RESOURCES

To learn more about use of low dose naltrexone in fibromyalgia and other conditions: www.lowdosenaltrexone.com.

Link to a current study on naltrexone in fibromyalgia: http://clinicaltrials.gov/ct2/show/NCT00568555?term=naltrexone+and +fibromyalgia&rank=2, accessed Feb 2010.

www.xyrem.com

16

ARE FIBROMYALGIA AND CHRONIC FATIGUE SYNDROME THE SAME DISEASE?

Doctors and patients alike are confused by the similarities between chronic fatigue syndrome (CFS) and fibromyalgia (FM). Current popular and medical opinion is that these conditions are actually the same illness. This is understandable since both are poorly understood conditions that are characterized by fatigue and primarily affect women.

Confusing matters further, the terms fibromyalgia and chronic fatigue syndrome are often used interchangeably or lumped together and treated as if they were the same disease. In fact, Dr. Jacob Teitelbaum, in his popular book *From Fatigued to Fantastic*, writes, "Chronic fatigue syndrome and fibromyalgia are the same illness in most cases." Throughout the book he uses the term CFS to refer to both fibromyalgia and chronic fatigue syndrome.[1]

Many of my fibromyalgia patients tell me they think they must have chronic fatigue syndrome because they feel fatigued all the time, and I think that is a common misperception. But there are actually very specific criteria to diagnose CFS, and it has a unique symptom profile and different triggers, and responds to different treatments than fibromyalgia. The fatigue in fibromyalgia appears to be from an entirely different source than in chronic fatigue syndrome.

The recent discovery of an unusual virus in the blood of CFS patients has lent support to the theory that CFS is a viral illness, whereas fibromyalgia is known to be due to dysfunction in the stress-response and processing of pain. It is of course possible for one person to have both fibromyalgia and chronic fatigue syndrome, but this is relatively rare in my experience.

While there are some overlapping symptoms, such as fatigue and muscle aches, there are distinct differences between these two conditions. Most CFS patients describe a sudden onset to their symptoms, often after a flu-like illness, suggesting that an infection triggers this syndrome. The ongoing symptoms of fatigue, low-grade fevers, sore throat, and swollen lymph nodes also suggest the presence of an infection. According to one medical review paper, "A severe flu-like illness occurs in most cases of chronic fatigue syndrome (CFS), suggesting that an infection triggers and possibly perpetuates this syndrome."[2]

Fibromyalgia, on the other hand, usually has a gradual onset, and is not associated with fevers, sore throats, or lymph node swelling.

For the past 30 years, many researchers have theorized that CFS is caused by a virus. There are certain telltale changes in the blood and immune cells when the body is fighting viral infections that are seen in patients with CFS. It has also been called "chronic mononucleosis syndrome" and "myalgic encephalomyelitis," both names reflecting the assumption that the cause was a viral infection.

But until recently, no one has been able to identify a specific virus associated with CFS. There were lots of false leads, including Epstein-Barr virus (EBV) and human herpes virus type 6 (HHV-6), but ultimately there was no convincing evidence linking these to CFS.[3]

Recently, however, a groundbreaking study isolated a specific virus in the blood of CFS sufferers. This study, published in the journal *Science* in 2009 and also covered in *The New York Times*, found that most chronic fatigue subjects tested positive for xenotropic murine leukemia virus-related virus (XMRV), compared to only 3.7 percent of healthy people. XMRV is a retrovirus, a member of the same family of viruses as the AIDS virus.[4]

I have long suspected chronic fatigue syndrome to have a viral cause. It often has a sudden onset and then can disappear as rapidly as it began. A close friend of mine developed chronic fatigue syndrome in college. She was extremely healthy and active on a competitive sailing team, until one day she suddenly came down with a severe flu-like illness. For six years she suffered crippling fatigue, dizziness, and foggy thinking. She stopped sailing and had to change her entire life to accommodate the 16-plus hours of sleep she needed each day just to function. And then one day, six years later, her illness completely resolved, just as suddenly and mysteriously as it began. She is now back to sailing and completely healthy. Throughout her illness, pain was not a huge issue, except for occasional muscle aches she described as similar to having the flu.

The onset of fibromyalgia tends to be much slower and more gradual, and is more often associated with a trauma such as a car accident. And there is no evidence of a viral infection in the blood in fibromyalgia. In fact, a study of the anti-viral medication acyclovir in fibromyalgia showed no reduction in symptoms.[5]

However, antivirals have shown some benefit in CFS. Two small studies of the antiviral drugs valcyclovir and gancyclovir found slight symptom improvement in CFS.[6, 7] In another study, seven of 10 patients treated with ribavirin, a broad spectrum antiviral with some activity against retroviruses, noted significant symptom improvement while on therapy, and relapse after stopping the medication.[8] Another drug, interferon, that stimulates the immune system to fight against all types of viruses, has shown mild benefit in CFS symptoms.[9, 10]

The antiviral drug poly(I)-poly(C)12U (Ampligen), which has specific activity against retroviruses, was shown to significantly improve CFS symptoms. A large, high-quality study with 24 weeks of this antiviral therapy resulted in increased energy, exercise tolerance, and cognitive functioning in CFS patients compared to those receiving placebo.[11]

Differences between chronic fatigue syndrome and fibromyalgia

While both illnesses primarily affect women, CFS is much less common than fibromyalgia. Whereas an estimated 2–3 percent of the American population has fibromyalgia, less than 0.2 percent is thought to have CFS.[12]

The diagnostic criteria to diagnose CFS include prolonged fatigue, sore throat, tender lymph nodes, and muscle pain.[13] (See text box on next page for further details.)

IN ORDER TO BE DIAGNOSED WITH CFS

YOU MUST HAVE:

1. Clinically unexplained fatigue of 6 months duration, that is not alleviated by rest and results in substantial reduction in previous levels of activities.

2. AND 4 or more of the following symptoms:

   - sore throat

   - tender lymph nodes in the neck or armpit

   - muscle pain

   - joint pain without swelling or redness

   - headache of a new pattern or severity

   - unrefreshing sleep

   - post-exertional malaise (fatigue) lasting greater than 24 hours

   - self-reported impairment in short-term memory or concentration

Certainly, anyone with fibromyalgia will recognize some of their symptoms on this list, especially muscle pain, fatigue, and non-refreshing sleep. But while it is very rare for a fibromyalgia patient to describe sore throat or tender lymph nodes, most patients with CFS do; 85 percent of patients with CFS complain of sore throat, 80 percent complain of swollen and tender lymph nodes, and 75 percent experience fevers.[14] Some researchers have even suggested that "symptoms of painful glands or fever might serve as clinical indicators distinguishing between fibromyalgia and the chronic fatigue syndrome."[15]

There are many other findings that support that CFS and fibromyalgia are different disorders in spite of overlapping symptoms. Substance P (a chemical important in the transmission of pain signals in the spinal cord) is quite elevated in the spinal fluid in fibromyalgia, but normal in CFS.[16] In fact, while some CFS patients will describe some muscle aches, the pain is usually described as minor. Fibromyalgia pain, in contrast, is more severe and is usually the primary issue.

While many studies have shown low growth hormone levels in fibromyalgia (as described in chapter 3), in CFS studies have found either normal or high growth hormone levels. Also, fibromyalgia patients have notable improvement in pain and tender points when given growth hormone injections, but CFS patients do not.[17, 18] Sodium oxybate (Xyrem), a medication that increases deep sleep, has shown significant symptom improvement in fibromyalgia, but not in CFS.[19]

Differences between CFS and FM

Chronic fatigue syndrome	Fibromyalgia
Symptoms begin suddenly with onset of flu-like symptoms and viral illness	Symptoms begin gradually
Onset not related to trauma	Onset usually related to trauma
Along with fatigue, most patients complain of sore throat, swollen lymph nodes and low-grade fever	Along with fatigue, most patients complain of muscle pain and stiffness
Responds to antiviral medications	Does not respond to antiviral medications
Normal growth hormone levels	Low growth hormone levels
Normal substance P levels in spinal cord	Elevated substance P in spinal cord, indicating abnormal pain processing
No symptom improvement with medication to induce deep sleep (sodium oxybate)	Symptoms improve with medication to induce deep sleep (sodium oxybate)

Of course, more research needs to be done to definitively prove that the XMRV virus causes CFS, but this is much stronger evidence supporting a viral cause to CFS then we have ever seen before. Studies to test whether antiretroviral drugs help in CFS will be an important next step, and likely a huge area of research in the next decade. I anticipate that as we gain more understanding of these two mysterious diseases, the differences between fibromyalgia and chronic fatigue syndrome will become even more apparent.

17

AN UNDERCOVER REPORT FROM MEDICAL TRAINING

I vividly remember sitting in clinic as a third-year medical student, when one of my fellow students picked up a big, thick patient chart and said: "Guess what this patient has? Fibromyalgia, of course!" This was greeted with sympathetic chuckles from the other students and doctors in the room.

I also remember a discussion I heard at a radiology conference during my fourth year of medical school. I was so disgusted by this interchange that I wrote it down word for word in my journal:

> The presenting doctor, discussing a vertebroplasty (putting cement into vertebrae to stabilize it after a compression fracture to reduce pain) that he had performed on a 53-year-old woman, said: "Well it didn't result in any improvement in pain, but I was tricked. No one told me she had fibromyalgia before I did the procedure."

> The audience chuckles and an older male doctor raises his hand and says, "I don't believe fibromyalgia exists."

> The presenter responded: "Well, that is a discussion for another day, but I am inclined to agree with you. In my

experience, patients with fibromyalgia don't get better until their lawsuit is resolved."

Which was greeted with more chuckling in the audience.

And these were some of the people that were grading me on my performance during medical school rotations! That is why I never told anyone in medical school that I had fibromyalgia.

Certainly, not all doctors are like this. I have had the pleasure to work with very dedicated, open-minded, and caring physicians and nurse practitioners who have devoted their career to studying and treating this illness.

Overall, though, it felt to me like fibromyalgia patients were viewed as whiners, as weaklings, as hopeless cases, and as a big no-reward drain on a doctor's time. I burned with anger when I heard the bashing of fibromyalgia patients, and part of me wanted to stand up and say: "Hey, I am one of *those people*. Look me in the eye and say that again!" But the grading system in medical training is highly subjective and based on the opinions of other students, residents, and supervising physicians, so I said nothing.

Instead I waited and plotted and wrote down what I heard them say about fibromyalgia. I often felt like I was undercover as a medical student. It was infuriating that one of my fellow students who was dealing with diabetes—meaning his pancreas did not function correctly—was looked at with admiration while I felt I had to keep the fact that my autonomic nervous system didn't function correctly as a deep, dark secret.

After my grades no longer mattered, I revealed that I had fibromyalgia to my colleagues and teachers during my final presentation at the end of my residency. I felt as if I was "coming out" and revealing a whole secret life. I felt I needed to show my fellow doctors that not only was fibromyalgia a real illness, but it could happen to one of them. And most importantly I wanted to show them that someone with fibromyalgia could get better and succeed even in a grueling and stressful career.

My colleagues were shocked, to say the least. As I have moved on in my career in clinical work and research, I have only selectively revealed that I have fibromyalgia, and for many of my current colleagues this book might be quite a surprise. I haven't even told my current primary care doctor that I have been seeing for five years, and he is a very good doctor. I just didn't want the dreaded scarlet letter "F" to be written in my chart.

A second-class diagnosis

A patient of mine described her surprise at how well she was treated by her medical team once she was diagnosed with breast cancer, as compared to when she was being treated for fibromyalgia. It seems to be regarded as a "second-class" diagnosis.

The complexities of this illness—along with the lack of diagnostic lab or imaging tests—have made for a particularly difficult relationship between Western medicine and fibromyalgia. The generally poor understanding of fibromyalgia among most doctors has also led, in my experience, to some unfortunate situations. If you are a woman of a certain age and you complain of pain to your doctor, you may very likely get a quick diagnosis of fibromyalgia without much workup. Once the word "fibromyalgia" appears in a patient's chart, almost any symptoms might be attributed to it without any further investigation.

A fibromyalgia patient was once referred to me by a primary care doctor due to worsening fatigue. He actually wrote in his notes, "She is in day 81 of a severe fibromyalgia flare, and so exhausted she was barely able to stand." In my exam room she looked pale and weak. Simple blood tests revealed she was severely anemic due to internal blood loss. Another patient of mine developed tremors, which her doctor attributed to fibromyalgia. I though this was odd, since fibromyalgia does *not* cause tremors, so I referred her to a neurologist who eventually diagnosed her with Parkinson's disease.

Diagnosing other problems in patients with fibromyalgia can be difficult because of the waxing and waning nature and a diverse array of symptoms. Patients themselves often attribute any source of pain and any new symptom to fibromyalgia. I say again and again to my patients that having fibromyalgia does not make you immune to getting other diseases that afflict humanity, such as diabetes, high blood pressure, or osteoarthritis.

Fibromyalgia results in muscle pain and fatigue, but does not affect the joints. So if you are having joint pain, it is probably due to osteoarthritis—also called "wear-and-tear" arthritis that affects every human body at some point in its life. Due to genetics and lifestyle, some people start getting osteoarthritis in their thirties, others not until their seventies. In every car, the brake pads will eventually wear out and need to be replaced, but some cars can make it many more miles until pads are so thin it causes problems. And unfortunately, in humans we can't actually replace our brake pads (the cartilage in our joints) so we all eventually end up with some amount of wear-and-tear arthritis.

Having fibromyalgia does not cause joint pain or arthritis, and it does not cause disk herniations in the spine. People with fibromyalgia can also have any number of other medical problems that can cause pain. So not all symptoms and not all pain are due to fibromyalgia. Unfortunately this means that even if your fibromyalgia symptoms improve, you might still have pain in your knees from arthritis, or numbness in your feet from diabetic neuropathy. But reducing central sensitization in fibromyalgia can help turn down the volume on any other pain signals, and in that way reduce all types of pain.

From the doctor's perspective

My anger and resentment toward doctors faded as I continued through medical training. The current medical system is just not set up well to deal with subtle and complex illnesses like fibromyalgia. There is too little time allotted to each patient, and too much dependence on quick fixes.

This is not entirely the fault of the medical profession. A lot of patients, myself included, come to the doctor and just want a quick fix, a pill that will make them feel better. Because there is no quick fix in fibromyalgia and we have had such limited tools in the toolbox for fibromyalgia, it can be a very frustrating experience for both patient and physician.

What I have realized in more than a decade of conventional medical training is that what is satisfying in the practice of medicine is figuring out the diagnosis, and seeing improvement with treatment. I often compare it to an auto-mechanic: He or she is trained to figure out what part of the car engine is broken, repair or replace that part, and get things running smoothly again. We are able to do that well for certain diseases: For example, the patient with carotid artery stenosis (clogging of one of the main vessels to the brain which can result in mini-strokes) whose symptoms completely resolve after physically operating on them and removing the clog.

But this is not the case with fibromyalgia. No wonder doctors are frustrated when dealing with an "engine" that is subtly malfunctioning, none of their diagnostic tests give them any leads, and all the treatments they try do little to help.

Fibromyalgia affects people from all across the socioeconomic spectrum, including those with advanced degrees like lawyers, MBAs, or engineers, as well as those with little education and no financial resources. Some people with fibromyalgia, as in the general population, also struggle with mental illness or addiction or poor coping skills. This minority of fibromyalgia patients has given the illness a negative reputation among doctors and in general society. The stigma associated with this illness leads many patients—myself included—to choose not discuss it with their doctor.

Certainly, as someone who has experienced this complex illness as both patient and physician, I have found that some fibromyalgia patients are emotionally exhausting to treat. But I have also taken care of difficult patients with other diseases, too, such as diabetes or high blood pressure. However, these conditions, unlike fibromyalgia, are easily understandable from a medical perspective. A patient that has both a poorly understood health condition like fibromyalgia combined with mental health issues can create a particularly challenging situation for any doctor.

Of course, the world of alternative medicine is not perfect either. There are way too many useless supplements and "cures" sold for fibromyalgia. Because people with fibromyalgia are so desperate for relief, they are easy prey for the snake-oil salesman. In particular there is a national chain of clinics focusing on fibromyalgia that offers expensive and complex hormone testing and treatment that is backed by very little science. I have had patients come to me after spending $15,000 on supplements and intravenous infusions at one of these clinics, and tell me that none of it helped.

I am not saying that all alternative therapies are bad. If they are effective I am absolutely in support of them. There may be some hormonal and IV therapies that are eventually shown to be helpful in fibromyalgia. And it is possible that the only patients that come to see me are those for whom those treatments did not work. But when there is scant evidence to support a therapy and patients tell me over and over that they don't find it helpful, it is hard for me to understand how they can charge such exorbitant prices.

In Chapter 14, I reviewed the available evidence for various alternative therapies to help you decide for yourself which are worth your money. And I encourage you to do your research on any alterative therapy before you spend thousands of dollars on it. In the reference section in the appendix, you can find instructions on how to research treatments using the same resources as doctors.

Ultimately the ideal treatment for fibromyalgia would utilize the best of alternative and Western medical care, based on therapies that have been shown to be helpful by clinical research. Also, a healthcare system where doctors are allowed more than 15 minutes per patient would help, but that is a subject for another entire book.

CONCLUSION

"Illness is not something to feel ashamed of. It is not a sign of misfortune or defeat. Suffering is the fuel of wisdom, and it opens the way to happiness. Through illness, human beings can gain insight into the meaning of life, understand its value and dignity, and strive to lead more fulfilling lives."
—Daisaku Ikeda

Medical science has learned so much about fibromyalgia in the past decade. It is a real and treatable illness. There are measurable scientific abnormalities in this illness and ways to effectively address most of them.

We don't yet have a cure, but we do have treatments that can help you feel much, much better. I predict that in the next decade, medical science will have fully figured out fibromyalgia, and it will be as accepted and treatable as diabetes—no longer treated as a second-class diagnosis.

My goal is to translate complex medical information into practical knowledge that people with fibromyalgia can use to get better. This is an ongoing process, and I will continue to learn more from patients, research studies, and my peers in healthcare. For the most recent updates, visit www.fridacenter.com.

I am done feeling ashamed that I have fibromyalgia. This illness has helped me to become a better doctor. My hyper-vigilant nervous system keeps me attuned to subtle changes in other people's emotional states and in my environment. And my intimate experiences with pain and suffering have made me a better human being.

Our lives should not be defined by our illnesses or diagnoses. Learn as much as you can about fibromyalgia and use the most effective therapies available. Then focus on living a bold and purposeful life, whatever that means to you.

ACKNOWLEDGEMENTS

To my patients—thank you for your trust in me.

I really appreciate the dedicated practitioners and researchers at Oregon Health and Science University who have inspired me and taught me so much about fibromyalgia, especially Kim Dupree Jones, Robert Bennett, and Cheryl Hyrciw.

I owe a debt of gratitude to the wonderful healers and teachers who helped me along the way, particularly Gisela Pikarsky, Yuliya Cohen, and Ben Benjamin.

Thank you to my reviewers and editors: Liz Liptan, Tracy Keenan Lloyd and Anne Michelle Graas. A big thank you to Allison Abell for her blunt (but brilliant) edits. The wise women of my life gave me hugely helpful advice, edits, and support: Merrilyn Tarlton, Jennifer Fay, and Kirsten Morgan.

My thanks to the staff at Legacy Pain Clinic for the good work they do (especially the best medical assistant in the world, Karan Serowik), and for understanding why I had to move on.

The support my family has shown me has been so wonderful. Mom, thanks for sticking around. Gina and JonPaul Fay, thanks for taking the leap with me.

This book would not have been possible without my husband's unconditional love and support. Jamie, you are the best editor, advisor, and husband a girl could ask for.

Finally, to Frida Kahlo, for inspiration. While struggling with chronic pain, she adorned herself with flowers, took the art world by storm, and attended her final art gallery showing being carried in her bed.

REFERENCES

A note about references:

For the majority of the references listed below, you can easily find the full article by going to www.pubmed.gov. This is an online database maintained by the United States National Library of Medicine that indexes most published research articles. The easiest way to find an article in this database is to enter the Pubmed PMID: an eight-digit number that identifies that specific article. You will find this number at the end of each reference listed below.

A small percentage of articles and journals are not indexed in this database, and the best way to find those is to search the lead author's last name and article title in a search engine like Google. If you still are not able to access it, a librarian at a medical school or teaching hospital can help you find articles. For some particularly important articles, I have included summaries and quotes from the articles that were too lengthy or detailed to include in the text.

Introduction: The F-word of Medicine

1. http://www.nytimes.com/2008/01/14/health/14pain.html?pagewanted=1&_r=1 accessed 7/1/10

2. Album D, Westin S. Do diseases have a prestige hierarchy? A survey among physicians and medical students. *Soc Sci Med.* 2008 Jan;66(1):182–88. PMID: 17850944

3. Bennett RM, Jones J, Turk DC, Russell IJ, Matallana L. An internet survey of 2,596 people with fibromyalgia. *BMC Musculoskelet Disord.* 2007 Mar 9;8:27. PubMed PMID: 17349056

Chapter 1: Overview of Fibromyalgia

1. Martínez-Lavín M, Amigo MC, Coindreau J, Canoso J. Fibromyalgia in Frida Kahlo's life and art. *Arthritis Rheum.* 2000 Mar;43(3):708–09. PMID: 10728769.

2. Bennett RM, Jones J, Turk DC, Russell IJ, Matallana L. An Internet survey of 2,596 people with fibromyalgia. *BMC Musculoskelet Disord.* 2007 Mar 9;8:27. PubMed PMID: 17349056

3. Veale D, Kavanagh G, Fielding JF, Fitzgerald O. Primary fibromyalgia and the irritable bowel syndrome: different expressions of a common pathogenetic process. *Br J Rheumatol.* 1991 Jun;30(3):220–22. PubMed PMID: 2049586

4. Wolfe F, Smythe HA, Yunus MB, Bennett RM, Bombardier C, Goldenberg DL, TugwellP, Campbell SM, Abeles M, Clark P, et al. The American College of Rheumatology 1990 Criteria for the Classification of Fibromyalgia. Report of the Multicenter Criteria Committee. *Arthritis Rheum.* 1990 Feb;33(2):160–72. PubMed PMID: 2306288

5. Bigatti SM, Hernandez AM, Cronan TA, Rand KL. Sleep disturbances in fibromyalgia syndrome: relationship to pain and depression. *Arthritis Rheum.* 2008 Jul 15;59(7):961–67. PubMed PMID: 18576297

6. Wolfe F, Clauw DJ, Fitzcharles MA, Goldenberg DL, Katz RS, Mease P, Russell AS, Russell IJ, Winfield JB, Yunus MB. The American College of Rheumatology preliminary diagnostic criteria for fibromyalgia and measurement of symptom severity. *Arthritis Care Res (Hoboken).* 2010 May;62(5):600–10. PubMed PMID: 20461783

7. Lawrence RC, Helmick CG, Arnett FC, Deyo RA, Felson DT, Giannini EH, Heyse SP, Hirsch R, Hochberg MC, Hunder GG, Liang MH, Pillemer SR, Steen VD, Wolfe F. Estimates of the prevalence of arthritis and selected musculoskeletal disorders in the United States. *Arthritis Rheum.* 1998 May;41(5):778–99. PubMed PMID: 9588729

8. White KP, Speechley M, Harth M, Ostbye T. The London Fibromyalgia Epidemiology Study: the prevalence of fibromyalgia syndrome in London, Ontario. J Rheumatol. 1999 Jul;26(7):1570–76. PubMed PMID: 10405947.

9. Arnold LM, Hudson JI, Hess EV, Ware AE, Fritz DA, Auchenbach MB, Starck LO, Keck PE Jr. Family study of fibromyalgia. *Arthritis Rheum.* 2004 Mar;50(3):944–52. PubMed PMID: 15022338

10. Middleton GD, McFarlin JE, Lipsky PE. The prevalence and clinical impact of fibromyalgia in systemic lupus erythematosus. *Arthritis Rheum.* 1994 Aug;37(8):1181–88. PMID: 8053957

11. "Fibromyalgia pain linked to brain dysfunction" in *Internal Medicine News* November 2009, 42(20): p. 21

12. Stockman R 1904 The causes, pathology and treatment of chronic rheumatism. *Edinburgh Medical Journal* 15: 107–16, 223-235

13. Gowers W 1904 Lumbago: its lessons and analogues. *British Medical Journal* 1: 117–21

Chapter 3: Fibromyalgia as a Chain Reaction

1. http://www.icnr.com/articles/thenatureofstress.html accessed Jan 2010

2. Martínez-Lavín M, Hermosillo AG, Rosas M, Soto ME. Circadian studies of auto-nomic nervous balance in patients with fibromyalgia: a heart rate variability analysis. *Arthritis Rheum.* 1998 Nov;41(11): 1966–71. PubMed PMID: 9811051

3. Furlan R, Colombo S, Perego F, Atzeni F, Diana A, Barbic F, Porta A, Pace F, Mal-liani A, Sarzi-Puttini P. Abnormalities of cardiovascular neural control and reduced orthostatic tolerance in patients with primary fibromyalgia. *J Rheumatol.* 2005 Sep;32(9):1787–93. PubMed PMID: 16142879

4. Torpy DJ, Papanicolaou DA, Lotsikas AJ, Wilder RL, Chrousos GP, Pillemer SR. Responses of the sympathetic nervous system and the hypothalamic-pituitary-adrenal axis to interleukin-6: a pilot study in fibromyalgia. *Arthritis Rheum.* 2000 Apr;43(4):872–80. PubMed PMID: 10765933.

5. Martínez-Lavín M, Hermosillo AG, Mendoza C, Ortiz R, Cajigas JC, Pineda C, Nava A, Vallejo M. Orthostatic sympathetic derangement in subjects with fibromyal-gia. *J Rheumatol.* 1997 Apr;24(4):714–18. PubMed PMID: 9101507.

> "In fibromyalgia there is a deranged sympathetic response to orthostatic stress. This abnormality may have implications regarding the pathogenesis of FM."

6. Bou-Holaigah I, Calkins H, Flynn JA, Tunin C, Chang HC, Kan JS, Rowe PC. Provocation of hypotension and pain during upright tilt table testing in adults with fibromyalgia. *Clin Exp Rheumatol.* 1997 May-Jun;15(3):239–46. PubMed PMID: 9177917.

> During tilt-table testing, 60 percent of patients with fibromyalgia exhibited an abnormal drop in blood pressure. Difficulty in maintaining blood pressure may contribute to symptoms of FM such as dizziness and fatigue.

7. Arnold LM, Hudson JI, Hess EV, Ware AE, Fritz DA, Auchenbach MB, Starck LO, Keck PE Jr. Family study of fibromyalgia. *Arthritis Rheum.* 2004 Mar;50(3):944–52. PubMed PMID: 15022338

8. Lutz J, Jäger L, de Quervain D, Krauseneck T, Padberg F, Wichnalek M, Beyer A, Stahl R, Zirngibl B, Morhard D, Reiser M, Schelling G. White and gray matter abnormalities in the brain of patients with fibromyalgia: a diffusion-tensor and volu-metric imaging study. *Arthritis Rheum.* 2008 Dec;58(12):3960–69. PubMed PMID: 19035484

9. Walker EA, Keegan D, Gardner G, Sullivan M, Katon WJ, Bernstein D. Psycho-social factors in fibromyalgia compared with rheumatoid arthritis: I. Psychiatric diagnoses and functional disability. *Psychosom Med.* 1997 Nov-Dec;59(6):565–71. PubMed PMID: 9407573

10. Amital D, Fostick L, Polliack ML, Segev S, Zohar J, Rubinow A, Amital H. Post-traumatic stress disorder, tenderness, and fibromyalgia syndrome: are they different entities? *J Psychosom Res.* 2006 Nov;61(5):663–69. PubMed PMID

11. Shin LM, Rauch SL, Pitman RK. Amygdala, medial prefrontal cortex, and hippocampal function in PTSD. *Ann N Y Acad Sci.* 2006 Jul;1071:67–79. Review. PubMed PMID: 16891563.

12. Romeo RD, Bellani R, McEwen BS. Stress-induced progesterone secretion and progesterone receptor immunoreactivity in the paraventricular nucleus are modulated by pubertal development in male rats. *Stress.* 2005 Dec;8(4):265–71. PubMed PMID: 16423715

13. Al-Allaf AW, Dunbar KL, Hallum NS, Nosratzadeh B, Templeton KD, Pullar T. A case-control study examining the role of physical trauma in the onset of fibromyalgia syndrome. *Rheumatology (Oxford).* 2002 Apr;41(4):450–53. PubMed PMID: 11961177

14. Greenfield S, Fitzcharles MA, Esdaile JM. Reactive fibromyalgia syndrome. *Arthritis Rheum.* 1992 Jun;35(6):678–81. PubMed PMID: 1599521

15. White KP, Speechley M, Harth M, Ostbye T. The London Fibromyalgia Epidemiology Study: the prevalence of fibromyalgia syndrome in London, Ontario. *J Rheumatol.* 1999 Jul;26(7):1570–76. PubMed PMID: 10405947

16. Holman AJ. Positional cervical spinal cord compression and fibromyalgia: a novel comorbidity with important diagnostic and treatment implications. *J Pain.* 2008 Jul;9(7):613–22. PubMed PMID: 18499527

17. Hryciw CA, Holman AJ. Positional cervical spinal cord compression as a comorbidity in patients with fibromyalgia (FM): findings from a one-year retrospective study at an FM referral university. *Myopain 2010, abstract 36*

18. Clauw DJ, Petzke F, Rosner MJ, Bennett RM. Prevalence of Chiari malformation and cervical spine stenosis in fibromyalgia. *Arth. Rheum.* 43: S173, 2000

19. Harding SM. Sleep in fibromyalgia patients: subjective and objective findings. *Am J Med Sci.* 1998 Jun;315(6):367–76. PubMed PMID: 9638893

20. Branco J, Atalaia A, Paiva T. Sleep cycles and alpha-delta sleep in fibromyalgia syndrome. *J Rheumatol.* 1994 Jun;21(6):1113–17. PubMed PMID: 7932424

21. Kooh M, Martínez-Lavín M, Meza S, Martín-del-Campo A, Hermosillo AG, Pineda C,Nava A, Amigo MC, Drucker-Colín R. Simultaneous heart rate variability and polysomnographic analyses in fibromyalgia. *Clin Exp Rheumatol.* 2003 Jul-Aug;21(4):529–30. PubMed PMID: 1294271.

Provides evidence that fight-or-flight hyperactivity at night is what causes the excessive arousal/awakening episodes and inability to get prolonged deep sleep.

22. Moldofsky H, Scarisbrick P, England R, Smythe H. Musculosketal symptoms and non-REM sleep disturbance in patients with "fibrositis syndrome" and healthy subjects. *Psychosom Med.* 1975 Jul-Aug;37(4):341–51. PubMed PMID: 169541

23. Felig, Phillip, Baxter JD, Frohman LA. *Endocrinology and Metabolism*, third edition. New York: McGraw Hill, 1995. p. 307.

24. Bagge E, Bengtsson BA, Carlsson L, Carlsson J. Low growth hormone secretion in patients with fibromyalgia—a preliminary report on 10 patients and 10 controls. *J Rheumatol.* 1998 Jan;25(1):145–48. PubMed PMID: 9458218

25. Leal-Cerro A, Povedano J, Astorga R, Gonzalez M, Silva H, Garcia-Pesquera F, Casanueva FF, Dieguez C. The growth hormone (GH)-releasing hormone-GH-insulin-like growth factor-1 axis in patients with fibromyalgia syndrome. *J Clin Endocrinol Metab.* 1999 Sep;84(9):3378–81. PubMed PMID: 10487713

26. Landis CA, Lentz MJ, Rothermel J, Riffle SC, Chapman D, Buchwald D, Shaver JL. Decreased nocturnal levels of prolactin and growth hormone in women with fibromyalgia. *J Clin Endocrinol Metab.* 2001 Apr;86(4):1672–78. PubMed PMID: 11297602

27. Paiva ES, Deodhar A, Jones KD, Bennett R. Impaired growth hormone secretion in fibromyalgia patients: evidence for augmented hypothalamic somatostatin tone. *Arthritis Rheum.* 2002 May;46(5): 1344–50. PubMed PMID: 12115242

28. Jones KD, Deodhar P, Lorentzen A, Bennett RM, Deodhar AA. Growth hormone perturbations in fibromyalgia: a review. *Semin Arthritis Rheum.* 2007 Jun;36(6):357–79. PubMed PMID: 17224178

29. Bennett RM. The origin of myopain: An integrated hypothesis of focal muscle changes and sleep disturbance in patients with the fibromyalgia syndrome. *Journal of Musculoskeletal Pain.* 1993; 1(3&4): 95–112.

30. Suh DY, Hunt TK, Spencer EM. Insulin-like growth factor-I reverses the impairment of wound healing induced by corticosteroids in rats. *Endocrinology.* 1992 Nov;131(5):2399–403. PubMed PMID: 1425438

31. Herndon DN, Hawkins HK, Nguyen TT, Pierre E, Cox R, Barrow RE. Characterization of growth hormone enhanced donor site healing in patients with large cutaneous burns. *Ann Surg.* 1995 Jun;221(6):649–56; discussion 656–59. PubMed PMID: 7794069

32. Bennett RM, Clark SC, Walczyk J. A randomized, double-blind, placebo-controlled study of growth hormone in the treatment of fibromyalgia. *Am J Med.* 1998 Mar;104(3):227–31. PubMed PMID: 9552084

33. Cuatrecasas G, Riudavets C, Güell MA, Nadal A. Growth hormone as concomitant treatment in severe fibromyalgia associated with low IGF-1 serum levels. A pilot study. *BMC Musculoskelet Disord.* 2007 Nov 30;8:119. PubMed PMID: 18053120

34. Gracely RH, Petzke F, Wolf JM, Clauw DJ. Functional magnetic resonance imaging evidence of augmented pain processing in fibromyalgia. *Arthritis Rheum.* 2002 May;46(5):1333–43. PubMed PMID: 1211524

35. Russell IJ, Orr MD, Littman B, Vipraio GA, Alboukrek D, Michalek JE, Lopez Y, MacKillip F. Elevated cerebrospinal fluid levels of substance P in patients with the fibromyalgia syndrome. *Arthritis Rheum.* 1994 37(11):1593–601. PubMed PMID: 7526868

36. Arendt-Nielsen L, Graven-Nielsen T. Central sensitization in fibromyalgia and other musculoskeletal disorders. *Current Pain and Headache Reports.*2003 7: 355–61

Chapter 4: Is Fibromyalgia Pain All In Your Spinal Cord?

1. Simms RW. Is there muscle pathology in fibromyalgia syndrome? *Rheum Dis Clin North Am.* 1996 May;22(2):245–66. PubMed PMID: 8860798

2. Bajaj P, Bajaj P, Madsen H, Arendt-Nielsen L. Endometriosis is associated with central sensitization: a psychophysical controlled study. *J Pain.* 2003 Sep;4(7):372–80. PubMed PMID: 14622679

3. O'Neill S, Manniche C, Graven-Nielsen T, Arendt-Nielsen L. Generalized deep-tissue hyperalgesia in patients with chronic low-back pain. *Eur J Pain.* 2007 May;11(4):415–20. PubMed PMID: 16815054

4. Kosek E, Ordeberg G. Abnormalities of somatosensory perception in patients with painful osteoarthritis normalize following successful treatment. *Eur J Pain.* 2000;4(3):229–38. PubMed PMID: 10985866

5. Bennett R. Fibromyalgia: present to future. *Curr Pain Headache Rep.* 2004 Oct;8(5):379–84. Review. PubMed PMID: 15361322

6. Starz TW, Vogt M, Gold K. 2008 Fibromyalgia: what's tender, what's not. *American College Rheumatology 2008 Annual Scientific Meeting, abstract 1405*

7. Staud R, Cannon RC, Mauderli AP, Robinson ME, Price DD, Vierck CJ Jr. Temporal summation of pain from mechanical stimulation of muscle tissue in normal controls and subjects with fibromyalgia syndrome. *Pain.* 2003 Mar;102(1–2):87–95. PubMed PMID: 12620600.

> Provides support for the role of painful input from the nerves of the muscles leading to the pain hyper-reactivity in fibromyalgia.

8. Staud R, Nagel S, Robinson ME, Price DD. Enhanced central pain processing of fibromyalgia patients is maintained by muscle afferent input: a randomized, double-blind, placebo-controlled study. *Pain.* 2009 Sep;145(1–2):96–104. PubMed PMID: 19540671.

> Injection of small amounts of lidocaine into a tender point in the trapezius muscle in fibromyalgia patients actually reduced the heightened sensitivity to heat in the skin of the forearm, completely away from the site of the injection. According to the article, central sensitization is "unlikely to occur in the absence of a pathological peripheral source or generator."

Chapter 5: Fascia Is the Source of Muscle Pain

1. Liptan GL. Fascia: A missing link in our understanding of the pathology of fibromyalgia. *J Bodyw Mov Ther.* 2010 Jan;14(1):3–12. PubMed PMID: 20006283

2. Gowers W 1904 Lumbago: its lessons and analogues. *British Medical Journal* 1: 117–21

3. Stockman R 1904 The causes, pathology and treatment of chronic rheumatism. *Edinburgh Medical Journal* 15: 107–16, 223–35.

4. Awad EA. Interstitial myofibrositis: hypothesis of the mechanism. *Arch Phys Med Rehabil.* 1973 Oct;54(10):449–53. PubMed PMID: 4126445

5. Grimm D. Biomedical research. Cell biology meets rolfing. *Science.* 2007 Nov 23;318(5854):1234–35. PubMed PMID: 18033859.

> An article about the first Fascia Research Congress in 2007 at Harvard University, a unique gathering of fascia researchers and bodyworkers.

6. Stecco C, Gagey O, Belloni A, Pozzuoli A, Porzionato A, Macchi V, Aldegheri R, De Caro R, Delmas V. Anatomy of the deep fascia of the upper limb. Second part: study of innervation. *Morphologie.* 2007 Mar;91(292):38–43. PubMed PMID: 17574469

7. Kellgren JH 1938 Observations on referred pain arising from muscle. *Clin Sci* 3:175–90

8. Bonica, J.J., 1990. *The Management of Pain.* Lea & Febinger, Philadelphia, p. 34.

> In fact most of the nerve endings in the muscle actually reside in the fascia 75 percent of the nerve endings in the muscle are actually in the fascia. Only 25 percent of the nerves connect to the muscle cells themselves.

9. Itoh K, Okada K, Kawakita K. A proposed experimental model of myofascial trigger points in human muscle after slow eccentric exercise. *Acupunct Med.* 2004 Mar;22(1):2–12; discussion 12-3. PubMed PMID: 15077932

10. Myllylä R, Salminen A, Peltonen L, Takala TE, Vihko V. Collagen metabolism of mouse skeletal muscle during the repair of exercise injuries. *Pflugers Arch.* 1986 Jul;407(1):64–70. PubMed PMID: 3016636

11. Armstrong RB, Ogilvie RW, Schwane JA. Eccentric exercise-induced injury to rat skeletal muscle. *J Appl Physiol.* 1983 Jan;54(1):80–93. PubMed PMID: 6826426

12. Yu JG, Malm C, Thornell LE. Eccentric contractions leading to DOMS do not cause loss of desmin nor fibre necrosis in human muscle. *Histochem Cell Biol.* 2002 Jul;118(1):29–34. PubMed PMID: 12122444

13. Tullson P, Armstrong RB. Muscle hexose monophosphate shunt activity following exercise. *Experientia.* 1981 Dec 15;37(12):1311–12. PubMed PMID: 7327240

14. Dodd JG, Good MM, Nguyen TL, Grigg AI, Batia LM, Standley PR. In vitro biophysical strain model for understanding mechanisms of osteopathic manipulative treatment. *J Am Osteopath Assoc.* 2006 Mar;106(3):157–66. PubMed PMID: 16585384

15. Schleip R, Klingler W, Lehmann-Horn F. Active fascial contractility: Fascia may be able to contract in a smooth muscle-like manner and thereby influence musculoskeletal dynamics. *Med Hypotheses.* 2005;65(2):273–77. PubMed PMID: 15922099.

> Some fibroblasts, in response to stress or strain, differentiate into myofibroblast, which are able to contract in a smooth muscle-like manner.

16. Stauber WT, Knack KK, Miller GR, Grimmett JG. Fibrosis and intercellular collagen connections from four weeks of muscle strains. *Muscle Nerve.* 1996 Apr;19(4):423–30. PubMed PMID: 8622719

17. Warhol MJ, Siegel AJ, Evans WJ, Silverman LM. Skeletal muscle injury and repair in marathon runners after competition. *Am J Pathol.* 1985 Feb;118(2):331–39. PubMed PMID: 3970143

18. Jarde O, Diebold P, Havet E, Boulu G, Vernois J. Degenerative lesions of the plantar fascia: surgical treatment by fasciectomy and excision of the heel spur. A report on 38 cases. *Acta Orthop Belg.* 2003 Jun;69(3):267–74. PubMed PMID:12879710

19. Snider MP, Clancy WG, McBeath AA. Plantar fascia release for chronic plantar fasciitis in runners. *Am J Sports Med.* 1983 Jul-Aug;11(4):215–19. PubMed PMID: 6614290

20. Kraushaar BS, Nirschl RP. Tendinosis of the elbow (tennis elbow). Clinical features and findings of histological, immunohistochemical, and electron microscopy studies. *J Bone Joint Surg Am.* 1999 Feb;81(2): 259–78. PubMed PMID: 10073590

21. Langevin HM, Stevens-Tuttle D, Fox JR, Badger GJ, Bouffard NA, Krag MH, Wu J, Henry SM. Ultrasound evidence of altered lumbar connective tissue structure in human subjects with chronic low back pain. *BMC Musculoskelet Disord.* 2009 Dec 3;10:151. PubMed PMID: 19958536

22. Bednar DA, Orr FW, Simon GT. Observations on the pathomorphology of the thoracolumbar fascia in chronic mechanical back pain. A microscopic study. *Spine.* 1995 May 15;20(10):1161–64. PubMed PMID: 7638659

23. Stauber WT, Clarkson PM, Fritz VK, Evans WJ. Extracellular matrix disruption and pain after eccentric muscle action. *J Appl Physiol.* 1990 Sep;69(3):868–74. PubMed PMID: 2123179

24. Mackey AL, Donnelly AE, Turpeenniemi-Hujanen T, Roper HP. Skeletal muscle collagen content in humans after high-force eccentric contractions. *J Appl Physiol.* 2004 Jul;97(1):197–203. PubMed PMID: 14990551

25. Koskinen SO, Wang W, Ahtikoski AM, Kjaer M, Han XY, Komulainen J, Kovanen V, Takala TE. Acute exercise induced changes in rat skeletal muscle mRNAs and proteins regulating type IV collagen content. *Am J Physiol Regul Integr Comp Physiol.* 2001 May;280(5):R1292–300. PubMed PMID: 11294746.

26. Spaeth M, Fischer P, Lagner C, Pongratz D 2005 Increase of collagen IV in skeletal muscle of fibromyalgia patients. *Journal of Musculoskeletal Pain* 12 (9S): 67.

Comparing specially stained muscle biopsies from 25 fibromyalgia patients to 26 healthy controls, they described an increase in collagen surrounding the muscle cells of the fibromyalgia patients.

27. Rüster M, Franke S, Späth M, Pongratz DE, Stein G, Hein GE. Detection of elevated N epsilon-carboxymethyllysine levels in muscular tissue and in serum of patients with fibromyalgia. *Scand J Rheumatol.* 2005 Nov-Dec;34(6):460–63. PubMed PMID: 16393769.

Increased levels of collagen in the fascia in fibromyalgia muscles, along with evidence for inflammation and tissue damage. Specifically, they note elevated levels of N-carboxymethyllsine (CML), an advanced glycation end-product (AGE) that is considered to be a marker of oxidative stress and tissue damage, in the fascia of fibromyalgia patients. "CML staining was stronger in the fibromyalgia patients, and was detected primarily in the interstitial tissue between the muscle fibers." They also reported increased staining of collagen types I, II, and VI in the fascia compared to healthy subjects and found "the collagens and CML were co-localized, suggesting that the AGE modifications were related to collagen." In addition, they found increased levels of CD-68 positive macrophages and activated NF-kB in the interstitial tissue of fibromyalgia muscles.

28. Miagkov AV, Kovalenko DV, Brown CE, Didsbury JR, Cogswell JP, Stimpson SA, Baldwin AS, Makarov SS. NF-kappa B activation provides the potential link between inflammation and hyperplasia in the arthritic joint. *Proc Natl Acad Sci U S A.* 1998 Nov 10;95(23):13859–64. PubMed PMID: 9811891.

NF-kB is a protein that plays an important role in the regulation of inflammation, and high levels of this protein are seen in joints inflamed due to rheumatoid arthritis.

29. Haslbeck KM, Friess U, Schleicher ED, Bierhaus A, Nawroth PP, Kirchner A, Pauli E, Neundörfer B, Heuss D. The RAGE pathway in inflammatory myopathies and limb girdle muscular dystrophy. *Acta Neuropathol.* 2005 Sep;110(3):247–54. Epub 2005 Jun 29. PubMed PMID: 15986224

30. Schleip R, Lehmann-Horn F, Klingler W 2006 Fascia is able to contract in a smooth muscle-like manner and thereby influence musculoskeletal mechanics. *Proceedings of the 5th World Congress of Biomechanics, Munich, Germany* : 51–54

31. Anders C, Sprott H, Scholle HC. Surface EMG of the lumbar part of the erector trunci muscle in patients with fibromyalgia. *Clin Exp Rheumatol.* 2001 Jul-Aug;19(4):453–55. PubMed PMID: 11491504

32. Bazzichi L, Dini M, Rossi A, Corbianco S, De Feo F, Giacomelli C, Zirafa C, Ferrari C, Rossi B, Bombardieri S. Muscle modifications in fibromyalgic patients revealed by surface electromyography (SEMG) analysis. *BMC Musculoskelet Disord.* 2009 Apr 15;10:36. PubMed PMID: 19368705

33. Kokebie R, Aggarwal R, Kahn S, Katz RS Muscle tension is increased in fibromyalgia: Use of a pressure gauge. *ACR abstracts* 2008 S 685

34. Schleip, R. Fascial plasticity- a new neurobiological explanation. Part 2. *Journal of Bodywork and Movement Therapies* 2003 7 (2):104–16

35. Anesini C, Borda E. Modulatory effect of the adrenergic system upon fibroblast proliferation: participation of beta 3-adrenoceptors. *Auton Autacoid Pharmacol.* 2002 Jun;22(3):177–86. PubMed PMID: 12452903

36. Oben JA, Yang S, Lin H, Ono M, Diehl AM. Norepinephrine and neuropeptide Y promote proliferation and collagen gene expression of hepatic myofibroblastic stellate cells. *Biochem Biophys Res Commun.* 2003 Mar 21;302(4):685–90. PubMed PMID: 12646223

37. Bhowmick S, Singh A, Flavell RA, Clark RB, O'Rourke J, Cone RE. The sympathetic nervous system modulates CD4(+)FoxP3(+) regulatory T cells via a TGF-beta-dependent mechanism. *J Leukoc Biol.* 2009 Dec;86(6):1275–83. PubMed PMID: 19741161

38. Murphy LJ, Vrhovsek E, Lazarus L. Identification and characterization of specific growth hormone receptors in cultured human fibroblasts. *J Clin Endocrinol Metab.* 1983 Dec;57(6):1117–24. PubMed PMID: 6313729

39. Oakes SR, Haynes KM, Waters MJ, Herington AC, Werther GA. Demonstration and localization of growth hormone receptor in human skin and skin fibroblasts. *J Clin Endocrinol Metab.* 1992 Nov;75(5):1368–73. PubMed PMID: 1430099

40. Gilpin DA, Barrow RE, Rutan RL, Broemeling L, Herndon DN. Recombinant human growth hormone accelerates wound healing in children with large cutaneous burns. *Ann Surg. 1994* Jul;220(1):19–24. PubMed PMID: 8024354

41. Herndon DN, Hawkins HK, Nguyen TT, Pierre E, Cox R, Barrow RE. Characterization of growth hormone enhanced donor site healing in patients with large cutaneous burns. *Ann Surg.* 1995 Jun;221(6):649–56; discussion 656–59. PubMed PMID: 7794069

Chapter 6: Causes of Inflammation

1. Katz RS, Kokebie R. Cytokine levels in fibromyalgia. Poster presented at 2008 American College of Rheumatology conference: accessed online (http://www.affter. org/affter_research/POSTER Katz_10-08_cytokines.pdf).

> Various serum cytokines including pro-inflammatory IL-6 were higher in fibromyalgia. "These suggest the possibility that inflammation and/or immune activity may contribute to symptoms in these patients."

2. Bazzichi L, Rossi A, Massimetti G, Giannaccini G, Giuliano T, De Feo F, Ciapparelli A, Dell'Osso L, Bombardieri S. Cytokine patterns in fibromyalgia and their correlation with clinical manifestations. *Clin Exp Rheumatol.* 2007 Mar-Apr;25(2):225–30. PubMed PMID: 17543146.

> Higher levels of IL-10, IL-8, and TNF-alpha were found in fibromyalgia patients compared to controls. "Our research suggests that chronic sub-inflammation and an impaired response of the immune system to stressors may be present in fibromyalgia." Interestingly, this study also showed that fibromyalgia patients with and without depression had similar cytokine levels; meaning it wasn't the depression causing the changes. Several cytokines can be elevated in depression, and some researchers have attributed elevated cytokine levels in fibromyalgia exclusively to depression.

3. Wang H, Moser M, Schiltenwolf M, Buchner M. Circulating cytokine levels compared to pain in patients with fibromyalgia, a prospective longitudinal study over six months. *J Rheumatol.* 2008 Jul;35(7):1366–70. PubMed PMID: 18528959.

Persistent elevation of IL-8 and TNF-alpha in fibromyalgia patients over 6 months. "Our results suggest that proinflammatory cytokines TNF-alpha and IL-8 are involved in FM, but they do not apparently provoke the pain of FM directly."

4. Kelley KW, Bluthé RM, Dantzer R, Zhou JH, Shen WH, Johnson RW, Broussard SR. Cytokine-induced sickness behavior. *Brain Behav Immun*. 2003 Feb;17 Suppl 1:S112–18. Review. PubMed PMID: 12615196

5. Gur A, Oktayoglu P. Status of immune mediators in fibromyalgia. *Curr Pain Headache Rep*. 2008 Jun;12(3):175–81. PubMed PMID: 18796266.

A very good review about inflammation in fibromyalgia, and notes the observation of fibromyalgia-like symptoms in patients treated for cancer with cytokine IL-2

6. Watkins LR, Maier SF. The pain of being sick: implications of immune-to-brain communication for understanding pain. *Annu Rev Psychol*. 2000;51:29–57. PubMed PMID: 10751964

7. Haack M, Sanchez E, Mullington JM. Elevated inflammatory markers in response to prolonged sleep restriction are associated with increased pain experience in healthy volunteers. *Sleep*. 2007 Sep 1;30(9):1145–52. PubMed PMID: 17910386.

Increased levels of IL-6 seen in healthy volunteers restricted to only four hours of sleep per night, who were also noted to have increased pain ratings. "Insufficient sleep quantity may facilitate and/or exacerbate pain through elevations of IL-6. In disorders where sleep disturbances are common, insufficient sleep quantity itself may establish and maintain its co-occurrence with pain and increased inflammation."

8. Goebel A, Buhner S, Schedel R, Lochs H, Sprotte G. Altered intestinal permeability in patients with primary fibromyalgia and in patients with complex regional pain syndrome. *Rheumatology (Oxford)*. 2008 Aug;47(8):1223–7. PubMed PMID: 18540025

9. Meddings JB, Swain MG. Environmental stress-induced gastrointestinal permeability is mediated by endogenous glucocorticoids in the rat. *Gastroenterology*. 2000 Oct;119(4):1019–28. PubMed PMID: 11040188

10. Kiziltaş S, Imeryüz N, Gürcan T, Siva A, Saip S, Dumankar A, Kalayci C, Ulusoy NB. Corticosteroid therapy augments gastroduodenal permeability to sucrose. *Am J Gastroenterol*. 1998 Dec;93(12):2420–25. PubMed PMID: 9860402

11. Bjarnason I, MacPherson A, Hollander D. Intestinal permeability: an overview. *Gastroenterology*. 1995 May;108(5):1566–81. PubMed PMID: 7729650

12. Panush RS. Food induced ("allergic") arthritis: clinical and serologic studies. *J Rheumatol*. 1990 Mar;17(3):291–94. PubMed PMID: 2332849

13. Karatay S, Erdem T, Yildirim K, Melikoglu MA, Ugur M, Cakir E, Akcay F, Senel K. The effect of individualized diet challenges consisting of allergenic foods on TNF-alpha and IL-1beta levels in patients with rheumatoid arthritis. *Rheumatology (Oxford)*. 2004 Nov;43(11):1429–33. PubMed PMID: 15304675

14. Randolph, Theron. Allergic Mylagia. *Journal of Michigan State medical society* 1951, 50:487–94

15. Bengtsson U, Nilsson-Balknäs U, Hanson LA, Ahlstedt S. Double blind, placebo controlled food reactions do not correlate to IgE allergy in the diagnosis of staple food related gastrointestinal symptoms. *Gut.* 1996 Jul;39(1):130–35. PubMed PMID: 8881824

16. Deuster PA, Jaffe RM. A novel treatment for fibromyalgia improves clinical outcomes in a community-based study. *Journal of Musculoskeletal Pain* 6(2):133–49.

> At both three and six months, the treatment group felt substantially better. Specifically at six months, the treatment group described 50 percent less pain, 70 percent less depression, and 50 percent more energy compared to pre-treatment. The control group reported increased levels of pain and depression, and similar level of stiffness and energy as compared to the beginning of the study. Unfortunately, in this study they only measured the ELISA/ACT results in FM patients, so they were not able to compare those results to healthy normal volunteers. However, according to the author of the study, "Previous work in our laboratory indicates that healthy normal control subjects show only rare reactions, the most common being cow's milk, corn and butylated hydroxytoluene."

17. Kaartinen K, Lammi K, Hypen M, Nenonen M, Hanninen O, Rauma AL. Vegan diet alleviates fibromyalgia symptoms. *Scand J Rheumatol.* 2000;29(5):308–13. PubMed PMID: 11093597

18. Donaldson MS, Speight N, Loomis S. Fibromyalgia syndrome improved using a mostly raw vegetarian diet: an observational study. *BMC Complement Altern Med.* 2001;1:7. PubMed PMID: 11602026

19. Michalsen A, Riegert M, Lüdtke R, Bäcker M, Langhorst J, Schwickert M, Dobos GJ. Mediterranean diet or extended fasting's influence on changing the intestinal microflora, immunoglobulin A secretion and clinical outcome in patients with rheumatoid arthritis and fibromyalgia: an observational study. *BMC Complement Altern Med.* 2005 Dec 22;5:22. PubMed PMID: 16372904

Chapter 8: Practical Diet Advice for Fibromyalgia

1. Veale D, Kavanagh G, Fielding JF, Fitzgerald O. Primary fibromyalgia and the irritable bowel syndrome: different expressions of a common pathogenetic process. *Br J Rheumatol.* 1991 Jun;30(3):220–22. PubMed PMID: 2049586

2. FitzGerald MP, Anderson RU, Potts J, Payne CK, Peters KM, Clemens JQ, Kotarinos R, Fraser L, Cosby A, Fortman C, Neville C, Badillo S, Odabachian L, Sanfield A, O'Dougherty B, Halle-Podell R, Cen L, Chuai S, Landis JR, Mickelberg K, Barrell T, Kusek JW, Nyberg LM; Urological Pelvic Pain Collaborative Research Network. Randomized multicenter feasibility trial of myofascial physical therapy for the treatment of urological chronic pelvic pain syndromes. *J Urol.* 2009Aug;182(2):570–80. PubMed PMID: 19535099

3. Pimentel M, Wallace D, Hallegua D, Chow E, Kong Y, Park S, Lin HC. A link between irritable bowel syndrome and fibromyalgia may be related to findings on lactulose breath testing. *Ann Rheum Dis.* 2004 Apr;63(4):450–52. PubMed PMID: 15020342

4. Deuster PA, Jaffe RM. A novel treatment for fibromyalgia improves clinical outcomes in a community-based study. *Journal of Musculoskeletal Pain* 6(2):133–49

Chapter 9: Solving the Exercise Dilemma

1. Jones KD, Liptan GL. Exercise interventions in fibromyalgia: clinical applications from the evidence. *Rheum Dis Clin North Am.* 2009 May;35(2):373–91. Review. PubMed PMID: 19647149

2. Horne JA. The effects of exercise upon sleep: a critical review. *Biol Psychol.* 1981 Jun;12(4):241–90. PubMed PMID: 7041996

3. Gowans SE, deHueck A. Pool exercise for individuals with fibromyalgia. *Curr Opin Rheumatol.* 2007 Mar;19(2):168–73. PubMed PMID: 17278933

4. Jones KD, Horak FB, Winters-Stone K, Irvine JM, Bennett RM. Fibromyalgia is associated with impaired balance and falls. *J Clin Rheumatol.* 2009 Feb;15(1):16–21. PubMed PMID: 19125137

5. Nitz JC, Kuys S, Isles R, Fu S. Is the Wii Fit a new-generation tool for improving balance, health and well-being? A pilot study. *Climacteric.* 2009 Nov 12. PubMed PMID: 19905991

6. Clark RA, Bryant AL, Pua Y, McCrory P, Bennell K, Hunt M. Validity and reliability of the Nintendo Wii Balance Board for assessment of standing balance. *Gait Posture.* 2010 Mar;31(3):307–10. PubMed PMID: 20005112

7. Gusi N, Parraca JA, Olivares PR, Leal A, Adsuar JC. Tilt vibratory exercise improves the dynamic balance in fibromyalgia: A randomized controlled trial. *Arthritis Care Res (Hoboken).* 2010 Mar 16. PubMed PMID: 20235191

8. Bautmans I, Van Hees E, Lemper JC, Mets T. The feasibility of Whole Body Vibration in institutionalized elderly persons and its influence on muscle performance, balance and mobility: a randomized controlled trial. *BMC Geriatr.* 2005 Dec 22;5:17. PubMed PMID: 16372905

9. Furlan R, Colombo S, Perego F, Atzeni F, Diana A, Barbic F, Porta A, Pace F, Malliani A, Sarzi-Puttini P. Abnormalities of cardiovascular neural control and reduced orthostatic tolerance in patients with primary fibromyalgia. *J Rheumatol.* 2005 Sep;32(9):1787–93. PubMed PMID: 16142879

Chapter 10: Improving Sleep—How to Stop Sleeping With One Eye Open

1. Bigatti SM, Hernandez AM, Cronan TA, Rand KL. Sleep disturbances in fibromyalgia syndrome: relationship to pain and depression. *Arthritis Rheum.* 2008 Jul 15;59(7):961–67. PubMed PMID: 18576297

2. Branco J, Atalaia A, Paiva T. Sleep cycles and alpha-delta sleep in fibromyalgia syndrome. *J Rheumatol.* 1994 Jun;21(6):1113–17. PubMed PMID: 7932424

3. Moldofsky H. The significance of the sleeping-waking brain for the understanding of widespread musculoskeletal pain and fatigue in fibromyalgia syndrome and allied syndromes. *Joint Bone Spine.* 2008 Jul;75(4):397–402. PubMed PMID: 1845653

4. Kooh M, Martínez-Lavín M, Meza S, Martín-del-Campo A, Hermosillo AG, Pineda C,Nava A, Amigo MC, Drucker-Colín R. Simultaneous heart rate variability and polysomnographic analyses in fibromyalgia. *Clin Exp Rheumatol.* 2003 Jul-Aug;21(4):529–30. PubMed PMID: 12942716

5. Affleck G, Urrows S, Tennen H, Higgins P, Abeles M. Sequential daily relations of sleep, pain intensity, and attention to pain among women with fibromyalgia. *Pain.* 1996 Dec;68(2-3):363–68. PubMed PMID: 9121825

6. Moldofsky H, Scarisbrick P, England R, Smythe H. Musculosketal symptoms and non-REM sleep disturbance in patients with "fibrositis syndrome" and healthy subjects. *Psychosom Med.* 1975 Jul-Aug;37(4):341–51. PubMed PMID: 169541

7. Lentz MJ, Landis CA, Rothermel J, Shaver JL. Effects of selective slow wave sleep disruption on musculoskeletal pain and fatigue in middle-aged women. *J Rheumatol.* 1999 Jul;26(7):1586–92. PubMed PMID: 10405949

8. http://www.webmd.com/fibromyalgia/features/living-with-fibromyalgia-and-chronic-fatigue accessed Oct 2010

9. Hindmarch I, Dawson J, Stanley N. A double-blind study in healthy volunteers to assess the effects on sleep of pregabalin compared with alprazolam and placebo. *Sleep.* 2005 Feb 1;28(2):187–93. PubMed PMID: 16171242

10. Drewes AM, Andreasen A, Jennum P, Nielsen KD. Zopiclone in the treatment of sleep abnormalities in fibromyalgia. *Scand J Rheumatol.* 1991;20(4):288–93. PMID: 1925417.

11. Moldofsky H, Lue FA, Mously C, Roth-Schechter B, Reynolds WJ. The effect of zolpidem in patients with fibromyalgia: a dose ranging, double blind, placebo controlled, modified crossover study. *J Rheumatol.* 1996 Mar;23(3):529–33. PMID: 8832997.

12. Shaw IR, Lavigne G, Mayer P, Choinière M. Acute intravenous administration of morphine perturbs sleep architecture in healthy pain-free young adults: a preliminary study. *Sleep.* 2005 Jun 1;28(6):677–82 PMID: 16477954

13. Hindmarch I, Dawson J, Stanley N. A double-blind study in healthy volunteers to assess the effects on sleep of pregabalin compared with alprazolam and placebo. *Sleep.* 2005 Feb 1;28(2):187–93. PubMed PMID: 16171242

14. Murphy KD, Rose MW, Chinkes DL, Meyer WJ 3rd, Herndon DN, Hawkins HK, Sanford AP. The effects of gammahydroxybutyrate on hypermetabolism and wound healing in a rat model of large thermal injury. *J Trauma.* 2007 Nov;63(5):1099–107. PubMed PMID: 17993957

15. Scharf MB, Baumann M, Berkowitz DV. The effects of sodium oxybate on clinical symptoms and sleep patterns in patients with fibromyalgia. *J Rheumatol.* 2003 May;30(5):1070–4. PubMed PMID: 12734908

16. Moldofsky H, Inhaber NH, Guinta DR, Alvarez-Horine SB. Effects of sodium oxybate on sleep physiology and sleep/wake-related symptoms in patients with fibromyalgia syndrome: a double-blind, randomized, placebo-controlled study. *J Rheumatol.* 2010 Oct;37(10):2156–66. PubMed PMID: 20682669

17. Russell IJ, Perkins AT, Michalek JE; Oxybate SXB-26 Fibromyalgia Syndrome Study Group. Sodium oxybate relieves pain and improves function in fibromyalgia syndrome: a randomized, double-blind, placebo-controlled, multicenter clinical trial. *Arthritis Rheum.* 2009 Jan;60(1):299–309. PubMed PMID: 19116896

18. Spaeth M, Russell IJ, Perrot S, Choy E, Benson B, Wang YG, Lai C. The effects of sodium oxybate on multiple symptoms of fibromyalgia: results from two phase 3, randomized, double-blind, controlled trials. *Myopain 2010 abstract 39*

Chapter 11: Manual Therapy for Your Fascia

1. Braddom, RL. *Physical Medicine and Rehabilitation.* WB Saunders. Philadelphia: 1996 p. 443

2. Barnes, JF. Fibromyalgia. *PT Today* March 4, 1996

3. Schleip R 2003 Fascial Plasticity- a new neurobiological explanation: Part 2. *Journal of Bodywork and Movement Therapies* 7 (2): 104–16

4. Sucher BM. Myofascial manipulative release of carpal tunnel syndrome: documentation with magnetic resonance imaging. *J Am Osteopath Assoc.* 1993 Dec;93(12):1273–78. PubMed PMID: 8307807

5. Crawford JS, Simpson J, Crawford P. Myofascial release provides symptomatic relief from chest wall tenderness occasionally seen following lumpectomy and radiation in breast cancer patients. *Int J Radiat Oncol Biol Phys.* 1996 Mar 15;34(5):1188–89. PubMed PMID: 8600109

6. Gamber RG, Shores JH, Russo DP, Jimenez C, Rubin BR. Osteopathic manipulative treatment in conjunction with medication relieves pain associated with fibromyalgia syndrome: results of a randomized clinical pilot project *J Am Osteopath Assoc.* 2002 Jun; 102 (6), 321–25. PubMed PMID: 12090649

7. Brattberg G. Connective tissue massage in the treatment of fibromyalgia. *Eur J Pain.* 1999 Jun;3(3):235–44. PubMed PMID: 10700351

8. Stockman R 1904 The causes, pathology and treatment of chronic rheumatism. *Edinburgh Medical Journal* 15: 107–16 and 223–35

9. Langevin HM 2008 Potential role of fascia in chronic musculoskeletal pain ; in *Integrative Pain Medicine*, edited by Audette and Bailey, Humana Press

10. Ward RC 2003 *Foundations for Osteopathic Medicine.* Lippincott, Williams & Wilkins, Philadelphia p. 1158

11. Gehlsen GM, Ganion LR, Helfst R. Fibroblast responses to variation in soft tissue mobilization pressure. *Med Sci Sports Exerc.* 1999 Apr;31(4):531–35. PubMed PMID: 10211847

12. Schleip R 2003 Fascial Plasticity- a new neurobiological explanation: Part1. *Journal of Bodywork and Movement Therapies* 7 (1): 11–19

13. Cottingham JT, Porges SW, Richmond K. Shifts in pelvic inclination angle and parasympathetic tone produced by Rolfing soft tissue manipulation. *Phys Ther.* 1988 Sep;68(9):1364–70. PubMed PMID: 3420170

14. Schleip R 2003 Fascial Plasticity- a new neurobiological explanation: Part 2. *Journal of Bodywork and Movement Therapies* 7 (2): 104–16

15. Leblebici B, Pektaş ZO, Ortancil O, Hürcan EC, Bagis S, Akman MN. Coexistence of fibromyalgia, temporomandibular disorder, and masticatory myofascial pain syndromes. *Rheumatol Int.* 2007 Apr;27(6):541–44. PubMed PMID: 17096090

16. Balasubramaniam R, de Leeuw R, Zhu H, Nickerson RB, Okeson JP, Carlson CR. Prevalence of temporomandibular disorders in fibromyalgia and failed back syndrome patients: a blinded prospective comparison study. *Oral Surg Oral Med Oral Pathol Oral Radiol Endod.* 2007 Aug;104(2):204–16. PubMed PMID: 17482850

17. FitzGerald MP, Anderson RU, Potts J, Payne CK, Peters KM, Clemens JQ,Kotarinos R, Fraser L, Cosby A, Fortman C, Neville C, Badillo S, Odabachian L, Sanfield A, O'Dougherty B, Halle-Podell R, Cen L, Chuai S, Landis JR, Mickelberg K, Barrell T, Kusek JW, Nyberg LM; Urological Pelvic Pain Collaborative Research Network. Randomized multicenter feasibility trial of myofascial physical therapy for the treatment of urological chronic pelvic pain syndromes. *J Urol.* 2009 Aug;182(2):570–80. PubMed PMID: 19535099

18. Lukban J, Whitmore K, Kellogg-Spadt S, Bologna R, Lesher A, Fletcher E. The effect of manual physical therapy in patients diagnosed with interstitial cystitis, high-tone pelvic floor dysfunction, and sacroiliac dysfunction. *Urology* 2001 Jun;57(6 Suppl 1):121–22. PubMed PMID: 11378106

19. Travell JG, Simons DG. *Myofascial pain and dysfunction: the trigger point manual.* Baltimore: William and Wilkins, 1983.

20. Lavelle ED, Lavelle W, Smith HS. Myofascial trigger points. *Med Clin North Am.* 2007 Mar;91(2):229–39. PubMed PMID: 17321283

21. Rabago D, Best TM, Zgierska AE, Zeisig E, Ryan M, Crane D. A systematic review of four injection therapies for lateral epicondylosis: prolotherapy, polidocanol, whole blood and platelet-rich plasma. *Br J Sports Med.* 2009 Jul;43(7):471–81. PubMed PMID: 19028733

Chapter 12: Reducing the Fight-or-Flight Response

1. Gibson TH, O'Hair D. Cranial application of low level transcranial electrotherapy vs. relaxation instructions in anxious patients. *American Journal of Electromedicine* 1987. 4(1):18–21

2. Podzolkov VI, Mel'nikova TS, Suvorova IA, Churganova LIu, Starovoĭtova SP. [Cranial electrostimulation—a new nondrug method of treating the initial stage of hypertension]. *Ter Arkh.* 1992;64(1):24–7. Russian. PubMed PMID: 1523556

3. Heffernan M. The effect of a single cranial electrotherapy stimulation on multiple stress measures. *Townsend Letters for Doctors and Patients* October 1995 :60–65

4. Lichtbroun AS, Raicer MM, Smith RB. The treatment of fibromyalgia with cranial electrotherapy stimulation. *J Clin Rheumatol.* 2001 Apr;7(2):72–78; discussion 78. PubMed PMID: 17039098

5. Cork RC, Wood P, Ming C et al. The effect of cranial electrotherapy stimulation (CES) on pain associated with fibromyalgia. *The Internet Journal of Anesthesiology* 2004 8(2).

6. Weiss MF. The treatment of insomnia through the use of electrosleep: an EEG study. *J Nerv Ment Dis.* 1973 Aug;157(2):108–20. PubMed PMID: 4146811

7. Smith RB. The effects of cerebral electrotherapy on short-term memory impairment in alcoholic patients. *International Journal of Addiction* 1977 12:562–75

8. Smith RB. Cranial electrotherapy stimulation in the treatment of stress related cognitive dysfunction with an eighteen-month follow up. *Journal of Cognitive Rehabilitation.* 1999 17:14–18

9. Moskalenko YE, Kravchenko TI, Vainshtein GB, Halvorson P, Feilding A, Mandara A, Panov AA, Semernya VN. Slow-wave oscillations in the craniosacral space: a hemoliquorodynamic concept of origination. *Neurosci Behav Physiol.* 2009 May;39(4):377–81. PubMed PMID: 19340579

10. Cheng S, Jacobson E, Bilston LE. Models of the pulsatile hydrodynamics of cerebrospinal fluid flow in the normal and abnormal intracranial system. *Comput Methods Biomech Biomed Engin.* 2007 Apr;10(2):151–57. PubMed PMID: 18651281

11. Kao YH, Guo WY, Liou AJ, Hsiao YH, Chou CC. The respiratory modulation of intracranial cerebrospinal fluid pulsation observed on dynamic echo planar images. *Magn Reson Imaging.* 2008 Feb;26(2): 198–205. PubMed PMID: 17826939

12. Maes M, Mylle J, Delmeire L, Altamura C. Psychiatric morbidity and comorbidity following accidental man-made traumatic events: incidence and risk factors. *Eur Arch Psychiatry Clin Neurosci.* 2000;250(3):156–62. PubMed PMID: 10941992

13. Arnold LM, Hudson JI, Keck PE, Auchenbach MB, Javaras KN, Hess EV. Comorbidity of fibromyalgia and psychiatric disorders. *J Clin Psychiatry.* 2006 Aug;67(8):1219–25. PubMed PMID: 16965199.

14. Walker EA, Keegan D, Gardner G, Sullivan M, Katon WJ, Bernstein D. Psychosocial factors in fibromyalgia compared with rheumatoid arthritis: I. Psychiatric diagnoses and functional disability. *Psychosom Med.* 1997 Nov-Dec;59(6):565–71. PubMed PMID: 9407573

15. Cloitre M. Effective psychotherapies for posttraumatic stress disorder: a review and critique. *CNS Spectr.* 2009 Jan;14(1 Suppl 1):32–43. Review. PubMed PMID: 19169192

16. Wang C, Schmid CH, Rones R, Kalish R, Yinh J, Goldenberg DL, Lee Y, McAlindon T. A randomized trial of tai chi for fibromyalgia. *N Engl J Med.* 2010 Aug 19;363(8):743–54. PubMed PMID: 20818876

Chapter 13: Should I Take Supplements for Fibromyalgia?

1. Mouyis M, Ostor AJ, Crisp AJ, Ginawi A, Halsall DJ, Shenker N, Poole KE. Hypovitaminosis D among rheumatology outpatients in clinical practice. *Rheumatology* (Oxford). 2008 Sep;47(9):1348–51. Epub 2008 May 22. PubMed PMID:18499714

2. Tandeter H, Grynbaum M, Zuili I, Shany S, Shvartzman P. Serum 25-OH vitamin D levels in patients with fibromyalgia. *Isr Med Assoc J.* 2009 Jun;11(6):339–42. PubMed PMID: 19697583

3. Warner AE, Arnspiger SA. Diffuse musculoskeletal pain is not associated with low vitamin D levels or improved by treatment with vitamin D. *J Clin Rheumatol.* 2008 Feb;14(1):12–16. PubMed PMID: 18431091

4. Armstrong DJ, Meenagh GK, Bickle I, Lee AS, Curran ES, Finch MB. Vitamin D deficiency is associated with anxiety and depression in fibromyalgia. *Clin. Rheumatol.* 2007 Apr;26(4):551–54. Epub 2006 Jul 19. PubMed PMID: 16850115

5. Cannell JJ, Hollis BW, Zasloff M, Heaney RP. Diagnosis and treatment of vitamin D deficiency. *Expert Opin Pharmacother.* 2008 Jan;9(1): 107–18. PubMed PMID: 18076342

6. Eyles DW, Smith S, Kinobe R, Hewison M, McGrath JJ. Distribution of the vitamin D receptor and 1 alpha-hydroxylase in human brain. *J Chem. Neuroanat.* 2005 Jan;29(1):21–30. PubMed PMID: 15589699

7. Gombart AF. The vitamin D-antimicrobial peptide pathway and its role in protection against infection. *Future Microbiol.* 2009 Nov;4: 1151–65. PubMed PMID: 19895218.

8. Lappe JM, Travers-Gustafson D, Davies KM, Recker RR, Heaney RP. Vitamin D and calcium supplementation reduces cancer risk: results of a randomized trial. *Am J Clin Nutr.* 2007 Jun;85(6):1586–91. Erratum in: *Am J Clin Nutr.* 2008 Mar;87(3):794. PubMed PMID: 17556697.

9. Simopoulos AP. Omega-3 fatty acids in inflammation and autoimmune diseases. *J Am Coll Nutr.* 2002 Dec;21(6):495–505. Review. PubMed PMID: 12480795

10. Maroon JC, Bost JW. Omega-3 fatty acids (fish oil) as an anti-inflammatory: an alternative to nonsteroidal anti-inflammatory drugs for discogenic pain. *Surg Neurol.* 2006 Apr;65(4):326–31. PubMed PMID: 16531187

11. Liperoti R, Landi F, Fusco O, Bernabei R, Onder G. Omega-3 polyunsaturated fatty acids and depression: a review of the evidence. *Curr Pharm Des.* 2009;15(36):4165–72. PubMed PMID: 20041818.

12. Su KP, Huang SY, Chiu TH, Huang KC, Huang CL, Chang HC, Pariante CM. Omega-3 fatty acids for major depressive disorder during pregnancy: results from a randomized, double-blind, placebo-controlled trial. *J Clin Psychiatry.* 2008 Apr;69(4):644–51. PubMed PMID: 18370571.

13. Su KP, Huang SY, Chiu CC, Shen WW. Omega-3 fatty acids in major depressive disorder. A preliminary double-blind, placebo-controlled trial. *Eur Neuropsychopharmacol.* 2003 Aug;13(4):267–71 PubMed PMID: 12888186

14. Carney RM, Freedland KE, Rubin EH, Rich MW, Steinmeyer BC, Harris WS. Omega-3 augmentation of sertraline in treatment of depression in patients with coronary heart disease: a randomized controlled trial. *JAMA*. 2009 Oct 21;302(15):1651–57. PubMed PMID: 19843899.

15. Regland B, Andersson M, Abrahamsson L, Bagby J, Dyrehag LE, Gottfries CG. Increased concentrations of homocysteine in the cerebrospinal fluid in patients with fibromyalgia and chronic fatigue syndrome. *Scand J Rheumatol*. 1997;26(4):301–7. PubMed PMID: 9310111

16. Miller AL. The methylation, neurotransmitter, and antioxidant connections between folate and depression. *Altern Med Rev*. 2008 Sep;13(3):216–26. Review. PubMed PMID: 18950248

17. Kelly CB, McDonnell AP, Johnston TG, Mulholland C, Cooper SJ, McMaster D, Evans A, Whitehead AS. The MTHFR C677T polymorphism is associated with depressive episodes in patients from Northern Ireland. *J Psychopharmacol*. 2004 Dec;18(4):567–71. PubMed PMID: 15582924

18. Godfrey PS, Toone BK, Carney MW, Flynn TG, Bottiglieri T, Laundy M, Chanarin I, Reynolds EH. Enhancement of recovery from psychiatric illness by methylfolate. *Lancet*. 1990 Aug 18;336(8712):392–95. PubMed PMID: 1974941

19. Passeri M, Cucinotta D, Abate G, Senin U, Ventura A, Stramba Badiale M, Diana R, La Greca P, Le Grazie C. Oral 5'-methyltetrahydrofolic acid in senile organic mental disorders with depression: results of a double-blind multicenter study. *Aging* (Milano). 1993 Feb;5(1):63–71. PubMed PMID: 825747

20. Coppen A, Bailey J. Enhancement of the antidepressant action of fluoxetine by folic acid: a randomised, placebo controlled trial. *J Affect Disord*. 2000 Nov;60(2):121–30. PubMed PMID: 10967371

21. Jacobs AM. Remittive therapy in the management of symptomatic and nonsymptomatic diabetic neuropathy. *Vascular Disease Management* 2009;5(3):63–71

Chapter 14: Alternative Therapies in Fibromyalgia—What Helps and What Doesn't

1. Michalsen A, Riegert M, Lüdtke R, Bäcker M, Langhorst J, Schwickert M, Dobos GJ. Mediterranean diet or extended fasting's influence on changing the intestinal microflora, immunoglobulin A secretion and clinical outcome in patients with rheumatoid arthritis and fibromyalgia: an observational study. *BMC Complement Altern Med*. 2005 Dec 22;5:22. PubMed PMID: 16372904

2. Bombardier CH, Buchwald D. Chronic fatigue, chronic fatigue syndrome, and fibromyalgia. Disability and health-care use. *Med Care*. 1996 Sep;34(9):924–30. PubMed PMID: 8792781

3. Sueiro Blanco F, Estévez Schwarz I, Ayán C, Cancela J, Martín V. Potential benefits of non-pharmacological therapies in fibromyalgia. *Open Rheumatol J.* 2008;2:1-6. Epub 2008 Jan 24. PubMed PMID: 19088863

4. Alfano AP, Taylor AG, Foresman PA, Dunkl PR, McConnell GG, Conaway MR, Gillies GT. Static magnetic fields for treatment of fibromyalgia: a randomized controlled trial. *J Altern Complement Med.* 2001 Feb;7(1):53–64. PubMed PMID: 11246937

5. Colbert A, Markov M, Banerji M, Pilla A. Magnetic mattress pad use in patients with fibromyalgia: a randomized double-blind pilot study. *J Back Musculoskeletal Rehabil.* 1999;13(1):19–31

6. McMakin CR , Gregory WM, Phillips TM 2005. Cytokine changes with micro-current treatment of fibromyalgia associated with cervical spine trauma. *J Bodywork Move Ther* 9(3) :169–76

7. Gür A, Karakoc M, Nas K, Cevik R, Sarac J, Ataoglu S. Effects of low power laser and low dose amitriptyline therapy on clinical symptoms and quality of life in fibromyalgia: a single-blind, placebo-controlled trial. *Rheumatol Int.* 2002 Sep;22(5):188–93 PMID: 12215864

8. Gür A, Karakoç M, Nas K, Cevik R, Saraç J, Demir E. Efficacy of low power laser therapy in fibromyalgia: a single-blind, placebo-controlled trial. *Lasers Med Sci.* 2002;17(1):57–61 PMID: 11845369

9. Hopkins JT, McLoda TA, Seegmiller JG, David Baxter G. Low-Level Laser Therapy Facilitates Superficial Wound Healing in Humans: A Triple-Blind, Sham-Controlled Study. *J Athl Train.* 2004 Sep;39(3):223–29. PubMed PMID: 15496990

10. Simunovic Z, Trobonjaca T, Trobonjaca Z. Treatment of medial and lateral epicondylitis (tennis and golfer's elbow) with low-level laser therapy: amulticenter double blind, placebo-controlled clinical study on 324 patients. *J Clin Laser Med Surg.* 1998 Jun;16(3):145–51. PubMed PMID: 9743652

11. Lam LK, Cheing GL. Effects of 904-nm low-level laser therapy in the manage-ment of lateral epicondylitis: a randomized controlled trial. *Photomed Laser Surg.* 2007 Apr;25(2):65–71. PubMed PMID: 17508839

12. Saygun I, Karacay S, Serdar M, Ural AU, Sencimen M, Kurtis B. Effects of laser irradiation on the release of basic fibroblast growth factor (bFGF), insulin, like growth factor-1 (IGF-1), and receptor of IGF-1 (IGFBP3) from gingival fibroblasts. *Lasers Med Sci.* 2008 Apr;23(2):
211–15. Epub 2007 Jul 10. PubMed PMID: 17619941

13. Chen CH, Tsai JL, Wang YH, Lee CL, Chen JK, Huang MH. Low-level laser irradiation promotes cell proliferation and mRNA expression of type I collagen and decorin in porcine Achilles tendon fibroblasts in vitro. *J Orthop Res.* 2009 May;27(5):646–50. PubMed PMID: 18991342

14. Thorsen H, Gam AN, Svensson BH, Jess M, Jensen MK, Piculell I, Schack LK,Skjøtt K. Low-level laser therapy for myofascial pain in the neck and shoulder girdle. A double-blind, cross-over study. *Scand J Rheumatol.* 1992;21(3):139–41PubMed PMID: 1604252

15. Whelan HT, Smits RL Jr, Buchman EV, Whelan NT, Turner SG, Margolis DA,Cevenini V, Stinson H, Ignatius R, Martin T, Cwiklinski J, Philippi AF, Graf WR, Hodgson B, Gould L, Kane M, Chen G, Caviness J. Effect of NASA light-emitting diode irradiation on wound healing. *J Clin Laser Med Surg.* 2001 Dec;19(6):305–14 PubMed PMID: 11776448

16. Field T, Diego M, Cullen C, Hernandez-Reif M, Sunshine W, Douglas S. Fibromyalgia pain and substance P decrease and sleep improves after massage therapy. *J Clin Rheumatol.* 2002 Apr;8(2):72–76. PubMed PMID: 17041326

17. Brattberg G. Connective tissue massage in the treatment of fibromyalgia. *Eur J Pain.* 1999 Jun;3(3):235–44. PubMed PMID: 10700351

18. Gamber RG, Shores JH, Russo DP, Jimenez C, Rubin BR. Osteopathic manipulative treatment in conjunction with medication relieves pain associated with fibromyalgia syndrome: results of a randomized clinical pilot project. *J Am Osteopath Assoc.* 2002 Jun;102(6):321–25. PubMed PMID: 12090649

> A total of 24 patients were included in the study, and the treatment group received once weekly OMT sessions for 23 weeks. The control group received either moist heat packs at each visit or no additional treatment beyond their usual medications. The osteopathic manipulative techniques used in this study were individualized for each patient, so it is difficult to assess how much treatment directed specifically at the fascia that each patient received.

19. Unpublished study, www.myalgia.com.guaif2.htm

20. Tavoni A, Vitali C, Bombardieri S, Pasero G. Evaluation of S-adenosylmethionine in primary fibromyalgia. A double-blind crossover study. *Am J Med.* 1987 Nov 20;83(5A):107–10. PubMed PMID: 3318438

21. Jacobsen S, Danneskiold-Samsøe B, Andersen RB. Oral S-adenosylmethionine in primary fibromyalgia. Double-blind clinical evaluation. *Scand J Rheumatol.* 1991;20(4):294–302. PubMed PMID: 1925418

22. Russell IJ, Michalek JE, Flechas JD, Abraham GE. Treatment of fibromyalgia syndrome with Super Malic: a randomized, double blind, placebo controlled, crossover pilot study. *J Rheumatol.* 1995 May;22(5):953–58. PubMed PMID: 8587088

23. Ali A, Njike VY, Northrup V, Sabina AB, Williams AL, Liberti LS, Perlman AI, Adelson H, Katz DL. Intravenous micronutrient therapy (Myers' Cocktail) for fibromyalgia: a placebo-controlled pilot study. *J Altern Complement Med.* 2009 Mar;15(3):247–57. PubMed PMID: 19250003

24. Teitelbaum JE, Johnson C, St Cyr J. The use of D-ribose in chronic fatigue syndrome and fibromyalgia: a pilot study. *J Altern Complement Med.* 2006 Nov;12(9):857–62. PubMed PMID: 17109576

25. Finckh A, Berner IC, Aubry-Rozier B, So AK. A randomized controlled trial of dehydroepiandrosterone in postmenopausal women with fibromyalgia. *J Rheumatol.* 2005 Jul;32(7):1336–40. PubMed PMID: 15996074

26. Bennett RM, Clark SC, Walczyk J. A randomized, double-blind, placebo-controlled study of growth hormone in the treatment of fibromyalgia. *Am J Med.* 1998 Mar;104(3):227–31. PubMed PMID: 9552084

27. Cuatrecasas G, Riudavets C, Güell MA, Nadal A. Growth hormone as concomitant treatment in severe fibromyalgia associated with low IGF-1 serum levels. A pilot study. *BMC Musculoskelet Disord.* 2007 Nov 30;8:119. PubMed PMID: 18053120

28. Pamuk ON, Cakir N. The frequency of thyroid antibodies in fibromyalgia patients and their relationship with symptoms. *Clin Rheumatol.* 2007 Jan;26(1):55–59. PubMed PMID: 16541203

29. Bazzichi L, Rossi A, Giuliano T, De Feo F, Giacomelli C, Consensi A, Ciapparelli A, Consoli G, Dell'osso L, Bombardieri S. Association between thyroid autoimmunity and fibromyalgic disease severity. *Clin Rheumatol.* 2007 Dec;26(12):2115–20. PubMed PMID: 17487449

30. Lowe JC, Garrison RL, Reichman AJ, Yellin J, Thompson M, Kaufman D. Effectiveness and safety of T3 (triiodothyronine) therapy for euthyroid fibromyalgia: a double-blind placebo-controlled response-driven crossover study. *Clinical Bulletin of Myofascial Therapy* 1997, 2(2/3):31–58

31. Lowe JC, Reichman AJ, Yellin J. The process of change during T3 treatment for euthyroid fibromyalgia: a double-blind placebo-controlled crossover study. *Clinical Bulletin of Myofascial Therapy* 1997, 2(2/3):91–124

32. Kaartinen K, Lammi K, Hypen M, Nenonen M, Hanninen O, Rauma AL. Vegan diet alleviates fibromyalgia symptoms. *Scand J Rheumatol.* 2000;29(5):308–13. PubMed PMID: 11093597

33. Donaldson MS, Speight N, Loomis S. Fibromyalgia syndrome improved using a mostly raw vegetarian diet: an observational study. *BMC Complement Altern Med.* 2001;1:7. PubMed PMID: 11602026

34. Duester PA, Jaffe RM. A novel treatment for fibromyalgia improves clinical outcomes in a community-based study. *Journal of Musculoskeletal Pain* 1998; 6(2): 133–49

35. Jones KD, Liptan GL. Exercise interventions in fibromyalgia: clinical applications from the evidence. *Rheum Dis Clin North Am.* 2009 May;35(2):373–91. Review. PubMed PMID: 19647149

36. Gowans SE, deHueck A. Pool exercise for individuals with fibromyalgia. *Curr Opin Rheumatol.* 2007 Mar;19(2):168–73. PubMed PMID: 17278933

37. Wang C, Schmid CH, Rones R, Kalish R, Yinh J, Goldenberg DL, Lee Y, McAlindon T. A randomized trial of tai chi for fibromyalgia. *N Engl J Med.* 2010 Aug 19;363(8):743–54. PubMed PMID: 20818876

Chapter 15: Prescription Medications That Can Help

1. Hindmarch I, Dawson J, Stanley N. A double-blind study in healthy volunteers to assess the effects on sleep of pregabalin compared with alprazolam and placebo. *Sleep.* 2005 Feb 1;28(2):187–93. PubMed PMID: 16171242

2. Fibromyalgia: poorly understood; treatments are disappointing. *Prescrire Int.* 2009 Aug;18(102):169–73. PubMed PMID: 19746561

3. Clauw DJ. Pharmacotherapy for patients with fibromyalgia. *J Clin Psychiatry.* 2008; 69 Suppl 2:25–29. PubMed PMID: 18537460

4. Arnold LM. Biology and therapy of fibromyalgia. New therapies in fibromyalgia. *Arthritis Res Ther.* 2006;8(4):212. PubMed PMID: 16762044

5. Holman AJ, Myers RR. A randomized, double-blind, placebo-controlled trial of pramipexole, a dopamine agonist, in patients with fibromyalgia receiving concomitant medications. *Arthritis Rheum.* 2005 Aug;52(8):2495–505. PubMed PMID:16052595

6. Clark S, Tindall E, Bennett RM. A double blind crossover trial of prednisone versus placebo in the treatment of fibrositis. *J Rheumatol.* 1985 Oct;12(5):980–83. PubMed PMID: 3910836

7. Goldenberg DL, Felson DT, Dinerman H. A randomized, controlled trial of amitriptyline and naproxen in the treatment of patients with fibromyalgia. *Arthritis Rheum.* 1986 Nov;29(11):1371–77. PubMed PMID: 3535811.

8. Yunus MB, Masi AT, Aldag JC. Short term effects of ibuprofen in primary fibromyalgia syndrome: a double blind, placebo controlled trial. *J Rheumatol.* 1989 Apr;16(4):527–32. Erratum in: *J Rheumatol* 1989 Jun;16(6):855. PubMed PMID:2664173.

9. Tofferi JK, Jackson JL, O'Malley PG. Treatment of fibromyalgia with cyclobenzaprine: A meta-analysis. *Arthritis Rheum.* 2004 Feb 15;51(1): 9-13. PubMed PMID: 14872449

10. Vaerøy H, Abrahamsen A, Førre O, Kåss E. Treatment of fibromyalgia (fibrositis syndrome): a parallel double blind trial with carisoprodol, paracetamol and caffeine (Somadril comp) versus placebo. *Clin Rheumatol.* 1989 Jun;8(2):245-50. PubMed PMID: 2667860

11. Ware MA, Wang T, Shapiro S, Robinson A, Ducruet T, Huynh T, Gamsa A, Bennett GJ, Collet JP. Smoked cannabis for chronic neuropathic pain: a randomized controlled trial. *CMAJ*. 2010 Oct 5;182(14):E694–701. PubMed PMID: 20805210

12. Skrabek RQ, Galimova L, Ethans K, Perry D. Nabilone for the treatment of pain in fibromyalgia. *J Pain*. 2008 Feb;9(2):164–73. PubMed PMID: 17974490

13. Ware MA, Fitzcharles MA, Joseph L, Shir Y. The effects of nabilone on sleep in fibromyalgia: results of a randomized controlled trial. *Anesth Analg*. 2010 Feb 1;110(2):604–10. PubMed PMID: 20007734

14. Feinberg I, Jones R, Walker JM, Cavness C, March J. Effects of high dosage delta-9-tetrahydrocannabinol on sleep patterns in man. *Clin Pharmacol Ther*. 1975 Apr;17(4):458–66. PubMed PMID: 164314

15. Dussias P, Kalali AH, Staud RM. Treatment of fibromyalgia. Psychiatry (Edgmont). 2010 May;7(5):15-8. PubMed PMID: 20532153

16. Rao SG, Clauw DJ. The management of fibromyalgia. *Drugs Today (Barc)*. 2004 Jun;40(6):539–54. Review. PubMed PMID: 15349132

17. Furlan AD, Sandoval JA, Mailis-Gagnon A, Tunks E. Opioids for chronic non-cancer pain: a meta-analysis of effectiveness and side effects. *CMAJ*. 2006 May 23;174(11):1589–94. PubMed PMID: 16717269

18. Crofford LJ. Pain management in fibromyalgia. *Curr Opin Rheumatol*. 2008 May;20(3):246–50. PubMed PMID: 18388513

19. Sörensen J, Bengtsson A, Bäckman E, Henriksson KG, Bengtsson M. Pain analysis in patients with fibromyalgia. Effects of intravenous morphine, lidocaine, and ketamine. *Scand J Rheumatol*. 1995;24(6):360–65. PubMed PMID: 8610220

20. Harris RE, Clauw DJ, Scott DJ, McLean SA, Gracely RH, Zubieta JK. Decreased central mu-opioid receptor availability in fibromyalgia. *J Neurosci*. 2007 Sep 12;27(37):10000–6. PubMed PMID: 17855614

21. Shaw IR, Lavigne G, Mayer P, Choinière M. Acute intravenous administration of morphine perturbs sleep architecture in healthy pain-free young adults: a preliminary study. *Sleep*. 2005 Jun 1;28(6):677–82 PMID: 16477954

22. Bennett RM, Kamin M, Karim R, Rosenthal N. Tramadol and acetaminophen combination tablets in the treatment of fibromyalgia pain: a double-blind, randomized, placebo-controlled study. *Am J Med*. 2003 May;114(7):537–45. PubMed PMID: 12753877

23. Russell IJ, Kamin M, Bennett RM, Schnitzer TJ, Green JA, Katz WA. Efficacy of tramadol in treatment of pain in fibromyalgia. *J Clin Rheumatol*. 2000 Oct;6(5):250–57. PubMed PMID: 19078481

24. Younger J, Mackey S. Fibromyalgia symptoms are reduced by low-dose naltrexone: a pilot study. *Pain Med.* 2009 May-Jun;10(4):663–72. PMID: 19453963

25. Hutchinson MR, Zhang Y, Brown K, Coats BD, Shridhar M, Sholar PW, Patel SJ, Crysdale NY, Harrison JA, Maier SF, Rice KC, Watkins LR. Non-stereoselective reversal of neuropathic pain by naloxone and naltrexone: involvement of toll-like receptor 4 (TLR4). *Eur J Neurosci.* 2008 Jul;28(1):20–29. PMID: 18662331

26. McCleane G. Does intravenous lidocaine reduce fibromyalgia pain? A randomized, double-blind, placebo controlled cross-over study. *The Pain Clinic.* 2000; 12(3):181–185

> This randomized, double blind controlled study found that fibromyalgia pain scores reduced from an average of 7.3 (on a scale of 1–10) to 6.5 during the first week after lidocaine infusion, but did not reduce the use of pain medications over the following weeks. While the overall reduction in pain scores was not huge, some subjects had reductions in their pain of 50 percent or more. Of the 63 subjects tested, eight had more than 50 percent pain relief after the lidocaine infusion, while only one had that result after getting a placebo infusion. The pain scores slowly returned to baseline over the following three weeks.

27. Schafranski MD, Malucelli T, Machado F, Takeshi H, Kaiber F, Schmidt C, Harth F. Intravenous lidocaine for fibromyalgia syndrome: an open trial. *Clin Rheumatol.* 2009 Jul;28(7):853–55. PMID: 19263182

> This small study with no placebo group found that after 5 consecutive days of IV lidocaine infusion, pain scores reduced from 8.2 to 6.8, and at 30 days post infusion were still lower than before the lidocaine.

28. Raphael JH, Southall JL, Kitas GD. Adverse effects of intravenous lignocaine [lidocaine] therapy in fibromyalgia syndrome. *Rheumatology (Oxford).* 2003 Jan;42(1):185–56.PMID: 12509636

29. Hindmarch I, Dawson J, Stanley N. A double-blind study in healthy volunteers to assess the effects on sleep of pregabalin compared with alprazolam and placebo. *Sleep.* 2005 Feb 1;28(2):187–93. PubMed PMID: 16171242

30. Drewes AM, Andreasen A, Jennum P, Nielsen KD. Zopiclone in the treatment of sleep abnormalities in fibromyalgia. *Scand J Rheumatol.* 1991;20(4):288–93. PMID: 1925417.

31. Moldofsky H, Lue FA, Mously C, Roth-Schechter B, Reynolds WJ. The effect of zolpidem in patients with fibromyalgia: a dose ranging, double blind, placebo controlled, modified crossover study. *J Rheumatol.* 1996 Mar;23(3):529–33. PMID: 8832997.

32. Scharf MB, Baumann M, Berkowitz DV. The effects of sodium oxybate on clinical symptoms and sleep patterns in patients with fibromyalgia. *J Rheumatol.* 2003 May;30(5):1070–74. PubMed PMID: 12734908

33. Russell IJ, Perkins AT, Michalek JE; Oxybate SXB-26 Fibromyalgia Syndrome Study Group. Sodium oxybate relieves pain and improves function in fibromyalgia syndrome: a randomized, double-blind, placebo-controlled, multicenter clinical trial. *Arthritis Rheum.* 2009 Jan;60(1):299–309. PubMed PMID: 19116896.

34. Schwartz TL, Rayancha S, Rashid A, Chlebowksi S, Chilton M, Morell M Modafinil treatment for fatigue associated with fibromyalgia. *J Clin Rheumatol.* 2007 Feb;13(1):52. PubMed PMID: 17278955.

35. Schaller JL, Behar D. Modafinil in fibromyalgia treatment. *J Neuropsychiatry Clin Neurosci.* 2001 Fall;13(4):530–31. PubMed PMID: 11748325

Chapter 16: Are Fibromyalgia and Chronic Fatigue Syndrome the Same Disease?

1. Teitelbaum J. *From Fatigued to Fantastic.* Avery Trade. 3rd edition 2007, p.14

2. Chia JK. The role of enterovirus in chronic fatigue syndrome. J Clin Pathol. 2005 Nov;58(11):1126–32. PubMed PMID: 16254097

3. Lombardi VC, Ruscetti FW, Das Gupta J, Pfost MA, Hagen KS, Peterson DL, Ruscetti SK, Bagni RK, Petrow-Sadowski C, Gold B, Dean M, Silverman RH, Mikovits JA. Detection of an infectious retrovirus, XMRV, in blood cells of patients with chronic fatigue syndrome. *Science.* 2009 Oct 23;326(5952):585–89. PubMed PMID: 19815723.

4. http://www.nytimes.com/2009/10/09/health/research/09virus.html accessed 1/6/2010

5. Kendall SA, Schaadt ML, Graff LB, Wittrup I, Malmskov H, Krogsgaard K, Bartels EM, Bliddal H, Danneskiold-Samsøe B. No effect of antiviral (valacyclovir) treatment in fibromyalgia: a double blind, randomized study. *J Rheumatol.* 2004 Apr;31(4):783–84. PubMed PMID: 15088307

6. Lerner AM, Zervos M, Chang CH, Beqaj S, Goldstein J, O'Neill W, Dworkin H, Fitgerald T, Deeter RG. A small, randomized, placebo-controlled trial of the use of antiviral therapy for patients with chronic fatigue syndrome. *Clin Infect Dis.* 2001 Jun 1;32(11):1657–58. PubMed PMID: 11340544.

7. Lerner AM, Beqaj SH, Deeter RG, Fitzgerald JT. Valacyclovir treatment in Epstein-Barr virus subset chronic fatigue syndrome: thirty-six months follow-up. *In Vivo.* 2007 Sep-Oct;21(5):707–13. PubMed PMID: 18019402.

8. Chia JK. The role of enterovirus in chronic fatigue syndrome. *J Clin Pathol.* 2005 Nov;58(11):1126–32. Review. PubMed PMID: 16254097

9. See DM, Tilles JG. Alpha-interferon treatment of patients with chronic fatigue syndrome. Immunol Invest. 1996 Jan-Mar;25(1-2):153–64. PubMed PMID: 8675231

10. Brook MG, Bannister BA, Weir WR. Interferon-alpha therapy for patients with chronic fatigue syndrome. J Infect Dis. 1993 Sep;168(3):791–92. PubMed PMID: 8354926

11. Strayer DR, Carter WA, Brodsky I, Cheney P, Peterson D, Salvato P, Thompson C, Loveless M, Shapiro DE, Elsasser W, et al. A controlled clinical trial with a specifically configured RNA drug, poly(I).poly(C12U), in chronic fatigue syndrome. *Clin Infect Dis.* 1994 Jan;18 Suppl 1:S88–95. PubMed PMID: 8148460

12. Evengard B, Nilsson CG, Lindh G, Lindquist L, Eneroth P, Fredrikson S, Terenius L, Henriksson KG. Chronic fatigue syndrome differs from fibromyalgia. No evidence for elevated substance P levels in cerebrospinal fluid of patients with chronic fatigue syndrome. *Pain.* 1998 Nov;78(2):153–55. PubMed PMID: 9839828.

13. Fukuda K, Straus SE, Hickie I, Sharpe MC, Dobbins JG, Komaroff A. The chronic fatigue syndrome: a comprehensive approach to its definition and study. International Chronic Fatigue Syndrome Study Group. *Ann Intern Med.* 1994 Dec 15;121(12):953–59. PubMed PMID: 7978722.

14. Straus SE. The chronic mononucleosis syndrome. *J Infect Dis.* 1988 Mar;157(3):405–12. PubMed PMID: 2830340.

15. Wysenbeek AJ, Shapira Y, Leibovici L. Primary fibromyalgia and the chronic fatigue syndrome. *Rheumatol Int.* 1991;10(6):227–29. PubMed PMID: 2041979.

16. Evengard B, Nilsson CG, Lindh G, Lindquist L, Eneroth P, Fredrikson S, Terenius L, Henriksson KG. Chronic fatigue syndrome differs from fibromyalgia. No evidence for elevated substance P levels in cerebrospinal fluid of patients with chronic fatigue syndrome. *Pain.* 1998 Nov;78(2):153–55. PubMed PMID: 9839828

17. Bennett AL, Mayes DM, Fagioli LR, Guerriero R, Komaroff AL. Somatomedin C (insulin-like growth factor I) levels in patients with chronic fatigue syndrome. *J Psychiatr Res.* 1997 Jan-Feb;31(1):91–66. PubMed PMID: 9201651

18. Moorkens G, Wynants H, Abs R. Effect of growth hormone treatment in patients with chronic fatigue syndrome: a preliminary study. *Growth Horm IGF Res.* 1998 Apr;8 Suppl B:131–33. PubMed PMID: 10990148.

19. Scharf MB, Baumann M, Berkowitz DV. The effects of sodium oxybate on clinical symptoms and sleep patterns in patients with fibromyalgia. *J Rheumatol.* 2003 May;30(5):1070–74. PubMed PMID: 1273490

GLOSSARY

Acupuncture: a traditional Chinese method of healing using fine needles inserted at various points along the skin to affect body function.

Adrenaline: see *epinephrine*.

Allergen: a substance that causes an allergic reaction.

Allergic reaction: hypersensitive or pathological bodily reaction to a usually harmless substance.

Allopathic medicine: a system of medical therapy in which a disease or an abnormal condition is treated by medications or surgery to produce effects different from the disease or condition. Also called *Western medicine*. Most physicians in the U.S. currently practice this type of medicine.

Alpha-delta sleep: abnormal alpha wave (associated with wakeful states) intrusion into the delta waves of deep sleep.

Alternative medicine: any of the various systems of healing or treating disease that vary from Western medical standard practices (includes acupuncture, homeopathy, chiropractic, etc.). Also called *complementary medicine*.

Analgesic: a drug that relieves pain.

Anesthetic: any agent capable of producing anesthesia.

Anesthesia: a loss of sensation artificially produced by the administration of one or more agents that block the passage of pain impulses along nerve pathways to the brain.

Antigen: a substance, usually a protein, that the body recognizes as foreign and that can evoke an immune response.

Antibody: an immune protein produced by lymphocytes in response to bacteria, viruses and other antigenic substances. An antibody is specific to an antigen.

Antiviral drug: a medication directed against viruses.

Asthma: a chronic lung disorder marked by recurring episodes of labored breathing, wheezing, and coughing that are triggered by hyper-reactivity to various stimuli, such as allergens.

Atom: the smallest particle of an element. Atoms contain neutrons, electrons, and protons.

Autoimmune disease: a large group of diseases characterized by an alteration in the function of the immune system, resulting in antibodies against the body's own tissue. Examples include rheumatoid arthritis and lupus.

Autonomic nervous system: the part of the nervous system that regulates involuntary functions in the body, including the activity of the cardiac muscle, smooth muscles, and glands. It has two divisions: the sympathetic nervous system which accelerates heart rate, constricts blood vessels, and raises blood pressure; and the parasympathetic nervous system which slows heart rate, increases gland activity and movement in the digestive system

Benzodiazepine: a group of psychotropic medications that includes diazepam, lorazepam, and clonazepam that can reduce anxiety and induce sleep.

Candida albicans: a common yeast organism that normally lives in the mucous membranes of the mouth, intestinal tract, vagina, and skin of the human body.

Central nervous system: consists of the brain and spinal cord, and is the main network of coordination and control for the entire body.

Central sensitization: a state in which spinal cord neurons activated by noxious mechanical and chemical input from peripheral nerves are sensitized and become hyper-responsive to all subsequent signals from the nerves.

Collagen: fibrous protein that is the chief constituent of connective tissues such as tendons, ligaments, and fascia.

Connective tissue: a dense tissue that supports and binds together other body tissue. Contains large amounts of cells and intercellular material.

Corticosteroids: the group of hormones secreted by the adrenal glands that influence many functions of the body. Synthetic versions of these hormones are used as medications.

Crohn's disease: a chronic inflammatory bowel disease of unknown origin, characterized by diarrhea, cramping, weight loss, and local abscess formation and scarring.

Cytokines: proteins secreted by cells and used to communicate with other cells, especially cells of the immune system.

Double blind: an experimental procedure in which neither the subjects nor the experimenters know which subjects are in the experiment group and which are in the control group during the actual course of the experiments.

Endomysium: the delicate connective tissue surrounding individual muscle fibers (together with the epimysium and perimysium composes the fascia of the muscle).

Endorphins: chemicals produced by the brain that bind to opiate receptors and act as natural painkillers.

Enzyme-Linked ImmunoSorbent Assay/Advanced Cell Test (ELISA/ACT): a blood test that analyzes lymphocytes (immune blood cells) response to foreign invaders under controlled laboratory conditions as they react in the bloodstream, providing information about delayed allergies.

Epimysium: the external connective tissue sheet of the muscle (together with the endomysium and perimysium composes the fascia of the muscle).

Epinephrine: a hormone that is secreted by the adrenal glands as part of the sympathetic nervous system's response to stress, and is important in regulating body functions including blood pressure and heart rate. Also called *adrenaline*.

Extracellular matrix: a gel-like substance containing collagen, elastin, proteoglycans, and fluid. Produced by the cells embedded in the gel (the fibroblast produces the extracellular matrix of the connective tissue).

Fascia: a sheet of connective tissue covering or binding together body structures. See Chapter 5 for a discussion of the fascia as it relates to the muscle.

Fibrositis: a rheumatic disease affecting fibrous tissue. Also an old name for fibromyalgia.

Fibroblast: a connective-tissue cell that secretes the proteins and collagen that forms extracellular fibrillar matrix of the connective tissue.

Food and Drug Administration (FDA): U.S. federal agency responsible for the enforcement of federal safety regulations on the sale of food, drugs, and cosmetics.

Friction massage: a type of massage that uses manual pressure across a tendon to break up scar tissue and adhesions. Also called *cross-fiber friction massage*, *deep transverse friction*, or *friction therapy*.

Glia: cells of the nervous system that have a supportive function to neurons.

Growth hormone: a hormone secreted by the pituitary gland in the brain that has multiple effects on the body. In childhood it promotes linear growth, in adulthood it is important for tissue regeneration and healing.

High Efficiency Particulate Air (HEPA) filter: air filters designed to remove airborne pathogens.

Hormone: a chemical substance produced by cells in one part of the body that regulates the activity of cells in another part of the body.

Hypothalamus: a part of the brain that activates, controls, and integrates the peripheral autonomic system and many other body functions including temperature, sleep, and appetite.

Hypothesis: a statement derived from a theory that is tentatively assumed in order to test its consistency with facts that are known or may be determined.

Immune system: the bodily system that protects the body from foreign substances, cells, and tissues by producing the immune response and that includes the thymus, spleen, lymph nodes, special deposits of lymphoid tissue (as in the gastrointestinal tract and bone marrow), lymphocytes (including the B cells and T cells), and antibodies.

Immunomodulatory: a drug that modifies the immune response or the functioning of the immune system (as by the stimulation of antibody formation or the inhibition of white blood cell activity).

Inflammation: the protective response of body tissue to irritation or injury that may be acute or chronic, and is mediated by multiple chemical messengers including prostaglandins, histamine, and cytokines.

Infusion: the introduction of a substance such as a fluid, nutrient or drug directly into a vein.

Interstitial: the space between cells.

Intravenous: administered by entering a vein.

Ligament: white shiny bands of connective tissue that connect bone to bone and bind joints together.

Lupus (systemic lupus erythematosus): a chronic inflammatory connective tissue disease that affects many systems of the body and is characterized by skin rash, arthritis, anemia, and in serious cases by involvement of the kidneys and central nervous system. Also called *systemic lupus* or *SLE*.

Lymphocyte: a type of white blood cell that makes antibodies and is very important in the immune defense.

Magnetic Resonance Imaging (MRI): a medical imaging technique that uses radiofrequency radiation to create an image of internal body tissue.

Manual therapy: therapeutic touching or manipulation of the body by using one of many different specialized techniques. Also called *bodywork*.

Massage: manipulation of soft-tissue (by rubbing, kneading, or stroking) with the hand or and instrument for therapeutic purposes.

Myofascia: the fascia, or sheets of connective tissue, supporting and binding together the muscles.

Myofascial Release (MFR): manual therapy technique designed to break up fibrosis and adhesions in the fascia.

Myofascial trigger points: discrete, hyperirritable spots located in a taut band of skeletal muscle that produce pain locally and in a referred pattern.

Myofiber: a single elongated muscle cell. Also called a *muscle fiber* or *muscle cell*.

Nerve: bundles of impulse carrying fibers that carry signals between the brain and spinal cord and the other parts of the body.

Neuron: the basic nerve cell of the nervous system.

Neuropathy: pain in the nerves due to nerve damage or inflammation, most commonly due to diabetes. Usually a burning, stinging or "pins and needles" type of pain, and can be accompanied by loss of sensation. Also called *peripheral neuropathy*.

Neurotransmitter: a substance (such as norepinephrine) that transmits nerve impulses between nerve cells.

Nociceptor: a peripheral nerve ending that reacts to tissue injury by causing pain.

Norepinephrine: acts as a neurotransmitter in the brain and in the sympathetic nervous system, and acts as a hormone when released by the adrenal glands in response to stress.

Objective: pertaining to a phenomenon or clinical finding that is observed and perceptible to persons other than the affected individual.

Opiate: a narcotic drug (such as morphine, heroin, and codeine) containing or derived from opium that can induce sleep and alleviate pain by binding with opiate receptors in the brain.

Osteopathic Manipulative Treatment (OMT): a technique used by osteopathic physicians to recognize and correct structural problems using manual manipulation of the body.

Osteopathic medicine: a therapeutic approach to the practice of medicine that includes all the usual forms of medical therapy and treatment but places a greater emphasis on the relationship between organs and musculoskeletal function.

Perimysium: the connective tissue sheath that surrounds a bundle of muscle fibers (forms the fascia of the muscle together with the epimysium and endomysium).

Peripheral nervous system: the motor and sensory nerves outside the brain and spinal cord. Includes the autonomic nervous system.

Placebo: an inactive substance used especially in experimental studies to compare the effects of the inactive substance with the experimental drug.

Plantar fasciitis: inflammation involving the plantar fascia of the base of the foot and causing pain under the heel when walking or standing.

Prostaglandin: one of several potent unsaturated fatty acids that have hormone-like activity in the human body, and are particularly important in the process of inflammation.

Randomized controlled trial: a clinical trial in which the subjects are randomly distributed into groups that are either subjected to the experimental procedure (as in the use of a drug) or which serve as controls. Also called *randomized clinical trial*.

Radioallergosorbent Test (RAST): a blood test used to determine to what substances a person is allergic. It measures specific IgE antibodies to suspected or known allergens. IgE is the antibody associated with Type I allergic response which are immediate and obvious (best example is hayfever due to pollen).

Retrovirus: any of the family *Retroviridae* of single-stranded RNA viruses, including HIV (human immunodeficiency virus).

Rheumatism: a nonspecific term for musculoskeletal aches and pains from any cause.

Rheumatoid Arthritis (RA): a chronic autoimmune disease that is characterized by pain, stiffness, inflammation, swelling, and sometimes destruction of joints.

Rolfing: a technique of deep massage intended to help the realignment of the body's connective tissue. Also called *structural integration*.

Serotonin: a hormone that has a variety of effects in the body and acts as a neurotransmitter in the brain. Low levels of serotonin are often associated with depression.

Slow-wave sleep: a stage of deep, dreamless sleep characterized by slow delta-waves in the brain and a low level of autonomic activity. Also called *deep sleep*.

Serotonin Norepinephrine Reuptake Inhibitor (SNRI): a class of antidepressant medications that increase the levels of both norepinephrine and serotonin in the brain.

Selective Serotonin Reuptake Inhibitor (SSRI): a class of antidepressants that increase serotonin levels in the brain.

Subjective: that which arises within or is perceived by the individual, as contrasted with something that can be evaluated by objective standards.

Substance P: a neurotransmitter that is important in transmission of pain signals in the nervous system.

Tender points: specific sites where muscles attach to bone that are excessively painful upon moderate pressure. In fibromyalgia, 11 of 18 specified tender pints must be painful for a diagnosis.

Tendinitis: an inflammatory condition of a tendon, usually resulting from strain.

Tendon: a glistening white band of dense fibrous connective tissue that connects a muscle with bone, transmits the force which the muscle exerts, and is continuous with the fascia of the muscle.

Tennis elbow: inflammation and pain over the outer side of the elbow usually resulting from excessive strain on and twisting of the forearm. Also called *lateral epicondylitis*.

Theory: a working hypothesis that is considered probable based on experimental evidence.

Temporal Mandibular Joint (TMJ) syndrome: pain or tenderness in the jaw area. Symptoms can include headache, earache, neck, back or shoulder pain, limited jaw movement, or a clicking or popping sound in the jaw. Can be caused by dysfunction of the temporomandibular joint or jaw muscles. Also called *temporomandibular disorder*, *temporomandibular joint disorder*, and *TMD syndrome*.

Xenotropic Murine Leukemia Virus-Related Virus (XMRV): a type of retrovirus recently implicated in chronic fatigue syndrome.

INDEX